Dedication

For Kate Kraft, with deep appreciation for your leadership, support, insight, and patience throughout all stages of the Planning and Designing the Physically Active Community project and to the active living movement as a whole. It wouldn't have happened without you.

Acknowledgments

My thanks go to my coauthors for this report, Rich Killingsworth, Jason Corburn, Bruce Appleyard, AICP, and Tim Torma. Also to Katharine Hannaford, who collected and managed all the photos and artwork in this report while working as a research assistant at APA, and Elaine Robbins, a freelance writer in Austin, Texas, who updated and refined the case studies in Chapter 6.

I deeply appreciate the generous input and camaraderie of the following people, past and present, at the Robert Wood Johnson Foundation and the Active Living Program offices: Kate Kraft, Rich Killingsworth, Brad Kahn, Marla Hollander, Leslie Linton, James Sallis, and Sarah Strunk, as well as Valerie Rogers and Jessica Solomon from the National Association of County and City Health Officials.

Additional thanks go to the planners, public health officials, and other advocates in the field who participated in numerous training workshops, conferences, and generally gave this report and its attendant tasks a reality check, including Rajiv Bhatia, Andrew Dannenberg, Larry Frank, Robert Glandon, Gerrit Knaap, Kevin Krizek, Bill Lennertz, Carol MacLennan, Nadejda Mishovsky, Kevin Nelson AICP, Matt Raimi, AICP, Karen Roof, Bill Wilkinson, AICP, and Paul Zykovsky, AICP.

Most of the photos in this report were taken by Dan Burden and were downloaded from the image bank at pedbikeimages.org. Speaking for everyone who's ever given a presentation on active communities, Thank You! The Minnesota Design Center's image library was also of significant help.

Finally, I thank my former colleagues at APA: Bill Klein, AICP, Jim Hecimovich, Lisa Barton, Kristin Raman, Michael Davidson, Maureen Ford, and Mary Eysenbach for their patience and support in seeing this project through.

Marya Morris, AICP

Planning Active Communities

Marya Morris, aicp, General Editor

TABLE OF CONTENTS

CHAPTER 1

A New Alliance: Planners and
Public Health Advocates

By Marya Morris, AICP

Supporters of good planning and smart growth have a new ally—public health practitioners and advocates. In the mid- to late 1990s, noting the tremendous increase in the rate of obesity in Americans and the limited success of the medical profession's efforts to persuade people to change their eating habits and get regular exercise, public health policy makers and researchers turned their attention to factors in the built environment that affect peoples' eating habits and exercise habits. In particular, they are focusing on patterns of development at the neighborhood, communitywide, and regional level, as well as transportation mobility options. Researchers are asking, Is there a correlation between urban sprawl and obesity? Has our auto-dependent lifestyle made it difficult to be physically active? As we've become more efficient in how we work, eat, and get around, have we engineered healthy behaviors and physical activity out of our daily routines?

RESEARCH ON SPRAWL AND OBESITY

A major study reported in the September/October 2003 issue of the *American Journal of Health Promotion* examined the relationship between sprawl and physical activity, obesity, and morbidity. The study, conducted by planner Reid Ewing, AICP, and several CDC researchers showed that, as sprawl increases, so do the chances that residents will be obese or have high blood pressure. People living in the most sprawling counties are likely to weigh six pounds more than people in the most compact county and are more likely to be obese. The study also found that people in sprawling areas walk less, which researchers said may indicate that people in more sprawling areas have fewer chances to stay fit through routine physical activity. Distance, lack of sidewalks and other barriers keep them from walking to the store or other destinations. Access to the full study and a supplementary report exploring its implications are available at www.smartgrowthamerica. org. Other studies from the special issue of the *American Journal of Health Promotion* are available at www.healthpromotionjournal.com. Studies on this same topic from a special issue of the *American Journal of Public Health* (September 2003) are available at www.ajph.org.

This new emphasis on design and the pattern of community growth has spawned numerous research studies, policy analyses, debates, and, increasingly, direct action to address the health problems associated with obesity and being overweight. In 2007, health experts and policy makers now recognize that built environment factors may be as much of a cause or contributor to obesity as other factors that had been studied for years, such as genetics, nutrition, and socioeconomic factors that lead to unhealthy eating and inactivity.

Indeed, the growing epidemic of obesity makes it imperative to reexamine planning policy and implement practical, on-the-ground modifications to the built environment. According to the National Health and Nutritional Examination Survey (NHANES) in 2004, the percentage of American adults who are obese has doubled since 1980, from 15 percent in 1980 to 32 percent. The widely disseminated maps—which are shown in Chapter 2 of this report—depicting obesity trends in the 50 states illustrate the extent of the problem.

The health profession's focus on the effects of the built environment on the public's health and physical activity comes at an opportune time for planning. In a climate where smart growth initiatives are increasingly under attack and the realities of implementing smart growth have proved difficult at all levels of government, the health profession is a welcome new partner with whom planners can collaborate on educating and demonstrating the benefits of smart growth. Health professionals, including medical doctors, are now coming to the table to make the case for broadening transportation options, creating walkable neighborhoods, mixing land uses, creating open space, and greening cities, generally leveling the playing field between people behind the wheel and people on foot. With health at the table, the challenges communities face today in trying to plan for growth and change will, with hope, no longer be reduced to an oversimplified "pro growth" vs. "no growth" argument, which has hindered many balanced, sensible, smart growth efforts in the last decade.

That said, we have a long way to go before health and physical activity become a routine, well-accepted element or aspect to local plans and development regulations. Even in this current era of planning marked by greater awareness of and commitment to smart growth, very few comprehensive and functional (e.g., transportation, land use, trails) plans even mention health or physical activity as a basis for smart growth.

Also energizing the policy focus on active communities is the burgeoning number of advocacy groups pushing for changes in transportation spending, land development, street design, and traffic calming—all in an effort to make their communities safer and more walkable. Such groups have been instrumental, for example, in getting "safe routes to school" legislation introduced, educating the public about existing and potential opportunities for physical activity, implementing traffic calming plans on neighborhood streets, and engendering public support for pedestrian- and bicycle-friendly policies.

The current flurry of policy analyses and interdisciplinary research on the environmental barriers to physical activity and potential solutions to overcome them are helping to lay a solid foundation for change. But much more work is needed to determine which specific modifications to the built environment, or combinations thereof, will be most effective in reversing current health and obesity trends.

What are the current conditions in most jurisdictions that run counter to the goal of creating active communities? Here is a sampling that ranges from the very broad to the very specific:

- The perpetuation (through zoning and subdivision regulations) of low-density development (e.g., one dwelling unit per acre or less), which is not conducive to walking or bicycling and thus not conducive to incorporating activity into daily routines.

- The regulatory and market barriers to mixed-use developments and districts. Regulatory barriers include development standards that prohibit combining various land uses within a single building or in a zoning district and building codes that discourage adaptive reuse of older buildings. Market barriers include bankers' resistance to providing developers financing for any project that constitutes a fundamental departure from conventional subdivision, strip shopping center, or big-box retail development. Plus, trends in retail, office, and industrial development—such as the proliferation of big box retail stores— reflect the development industry's need to continually adapt and change to meet household shopping preferences to increase market share. In many instances, such adaptations do not fit with a community's smart growth objectives and the vision of its citizens.

- The vast majority of streets and street environments in American cities and towns are, by design, unsafe and even hostile toward anything except the automobile. Conventional street design and engineering aim for the safe and efficient movement of vehicles to the exclusion of most other objectives, such as sharing the right-of-way with pedestrians and bicyclists. In private developments, priority is given to the location and size of parking lots and around moving vehicles, while transit users and pedestrians are left to navigate their way through parking lots and moving vehicles.

- The lack of street connectivity is another problem. Isolated, single-use subdivisions with no direct connection to surrounding shopping areas, schools, or other destinations make it very difficult for people to walk to their destination, even if they choose to do so.

- Not all new subdivisions are required to include sidewalks on both sides of the street or to address safe routes to local schools and shopping areas for people who live in the subdivision. Even where a developer is required to install sidewalks, planners may waive such requirements in exchange for a development "amenity" unrelated to neighborhood walkability. It is also the case that developers argue about the costs sidewalks add to development. Even some neighbors may prefer the rural feel of a neighborhood without sidewalks. But in suburban settings, residential streets without sidewalks send a clear message: no one walks here. Planners need to recognize the health consequences of such trade-offs or what might seem a fairly inconsequential requirement.

HOW THIS REPORT WAS PREPARED

This report is a product of APA's "Planning and Designing the Physically Active Community" project. The project, which began in 2001, was sponsored by The Robert Wood Johnson Foundation (RWJF), the nation's leading private health care and health policy charitable organization. RWJF has also funded numerous other nongovernmental organizations in its effort to bring the public's attention to the effects the built environment has on the obesity epidemic. Programs and projects led by other RWJF grantees are described below.

The project focused on the characteristics of predominant development patterns—and the role planning and land development controls have had in promulgating such patterns—with regard to peoples' ability to incorporate physical activity into their daily routine. Specifically, the project looked at

Specifically, the project looked at how planning processes, development regulations, and methods of community participation and collaboration can be modified and used to ensure that physical activity is a significant goal underlying the plans, provisions, and negotiations that lay the foundation for development patterns in a community.

how planning processes, development regulations, and methods of community participation and collaboration can be modified and used to ensure that physical activity is a significant goal underlying the plans, provisions, and negotiations that lay the foundation for development patterns in a community.

The U.S. Surgeon General's 1996 report on Physical Activity and Health (CDC 1996) recommended that all adults participate in at least 30 minutes of moderate-intensity physical activity on most, and preferably all, days of the week. At the same time, it had become clear to health experts that efforts to persuade people to change their individual behaviors to increase their level of physical activity and decrease the incidence of overweight and obesity were not working. In fact, obesity and overweight had reached epidemic status. It was time to look at other possible contributing factors and potential solutions that would allow people to stay or become active.

Expert Symposium and Training Institute

In March 2002, APA convened a group of experts in the fields of public health, planning, transportation, and urban design to discuss the relationship between planning, community design, and physical activity. The experts helped us to frame the issues of the project so that we could arrive at the best approach to presenting information, ideas, and examples to planners about how health and physical activity are affected by community design. One outcome of the symposium was a list of guiding principles (see sidebar) that define active communities, both in terms of the desired end result in creating such communities and the means by which localities may achieve that result.

In November 2003, APA convened a Physical Activity Institute in Nashville with invited participants from both planning and public health agencies in five jurisdictions we had identified as being proactive in creating active community environments. Faculty with expertise in public health, transportation planning, bicycle and pedestrian planning, and a private land developer were on hand to comment on the approaches the six teams described.

The jurisdictions were:

- The City of Albuquerque, New Mexico;
- Ingham County, Michigan;
- the Winnebago Indian Reservation, Nebraska;
- the City of Nashville, Tennessee; and
- State of New Jersey Department of Transportation.

Prior to the Institute, representatives from each participating jurisdiction prepared a case statement describing:

1. how they get started on incorporating public health and physical activity objectives into plans and planning process;
2. the tools they were using for interdisciplinary collaboration;
3. design solutions they had developed for specific districts (e.g., station area development) or facilities (e.g., trails and bikeways); and
4. the data and information they used to support planning for physically active communities.

At the Institute, each team presented their case example and received feedback from their peers on their approach and on possible next steps. Four faculty people also made presentations at the Institute, including a county public health director, a bicycle and pedestrian planning advocate, an urban design and transportation consultant, and a housing developer.

Bibliography

From the start of the project and continuing until this report went to print, we collected studies, reports, articles from the popular media, and academic journals that address the relationship between community design and physical activity. We also collected local comprehensive plans, transportation plans, health plans, and bicycle and pedestrian plans, among other plan types, as well as local ordinances and design guidelines that address walkability, connectivity, and the appearance and function of the built environment as it relates to peoples' ability and inclination to walk or engage in physical activity. Aiding in the resources development was an existing bibliography prepared by Frank and Engelke (2000), "How Land Use and Transportation Impact Public Health: A Literature Review of the Relationship between Physical Activity and Built Form," and many other bibliographies and resource lists compiled by authors and organizations engaged in active living initiatives.

Physical Activity and Health as a Planning Concern:
Results from a National Survey

Despite the relative inattention in the past to the various relationships between land-use planning, health, and physical activity in plans, a survey APA conducted as part of its project indicates growing public and planning profession awareness of the need to reconnect the disciplines.

This survey, conducted by APA in 2003 of 1,000 city planners, explored the extent to which planners and the local officials in their jurisdictions recognize the impacts of plans and land-use controls on physical activity.

Inasmuch as new public policy at the local level derives from how the mayor, the city council, or other officials react to specific events, trends, or new information, it is clear local officials see they have a policy-making role in this area (Figure 1-1). Twenty-eight percent of respondents said local appointed and elected leaders in their jurisdiction regard the physical activity of residents as an important public policy issue. An additional 36 percent said officials regard it as an emerging issue.

To improve the built environment to encourage physical activity, local officials must recognize that community planning and design—including land use, development patterns, transportation choice, and neighborhood design—are all part of the solution. According to the survey, 25 percent of

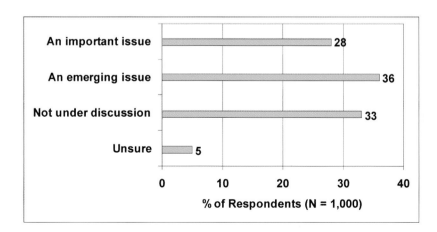

Figure 1-1. Responses of elected and appointed officials about the importance of residents' physical activity in their community.

Figure 1-2. Responses of elected and appointed officials about the relationship between community planning, design, and the ability of residents to engage in physical activity.

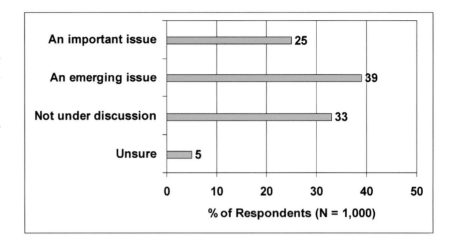

respondents reported that local officials did recognize the relationship between planning and public health, and another 39 percent said local officials' awareness of the relationship was emerging (Figure 1-2).

By their nature, comprehensive plans and land development regulations address a broad scope of community issues, including land use, housing, transportation, the environment, urban design, and economic development, among other elements. Despite the fact that approximately two-thirds (64 percent) of these plans recognize the importance of community planning and design as a key part of the solution, barriers remain to full incorporation of the explicit goal of promoting or allowing for physical activity in plans, projects, and regulations (Figure 1-3). The largest barrier, according to 40 percent of the respondents, is that physical activity is not yet regarded as a planning issue. The second greatest barrier (reported by 28 percent of respondents) is that physical activity is an assumed, not a stated, goal. Like most local government agencies, planning departments are perpetually faced with limited resources to tackle complex work programs and responsibilities. In that vein, 13 percent of respondents said the barrier to incorporating physical activity was that it would detract from other departmental priorities.

Figure 1-3. Barriers to incorporating physical activity goals and objectives in plans, projects, and regulations.

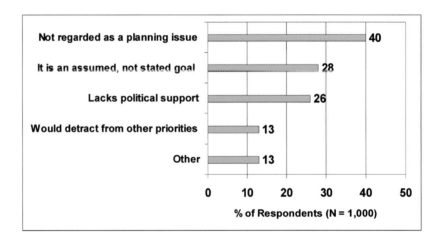

Next, APA asked planners which of the common types of plans in their jurisdiction contain *explicit* policies, goals, or objectives related to increasing physical activity opportunities for residents (Figure 1-4).

Based on the findings of other research APA has done on such plans, very few jurisdictions have such explicit policies. In this survey, however, many more respondents than expected said that several of their jurisdiction's plans contain such explicit policies. As shown in Figure 1-4, 64 percent indicated

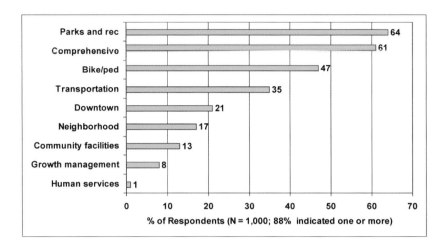

Figure 1-4. Activity-friendly planning undertaken by surveyed jurisdictions since 1998.

that the parks and recreation plan contains such explicit policies, 61 percent indicated that the comprehensive plan contains them, and 47 percent said the bicycle and pedestrian plan contains them.

A closer examination of the actual plan documents in question revealed that most plans did not contain specific policies. Respondents were most likely characterizing any policies, goals, and objectives related to walkability, alternate transportation modes, and quality of life enhancement—all of which are commonly found in the plans listed in the survey—as explicitly directed at increasing the physical activity levels of residents. While it is significant that planners *perceive* that physical activity and health of residents is being addressed in these plans, expressly stating such goals would be a stronger commitment to health on the part of the local jurisdiction and would result in programming and resources being directed at creating active communities. And, of course, broadening plans and the plan-making process to include health issues could help leverage substantial and previously untapped support for smart growth reforms jurisdictions have undertaken or will be undertaking. A similiar survey conducted in 2004 of APA and NACCHO members asked the same question but clairified that we were looking for plans that use the words "health" or "physical activity" explicitly.

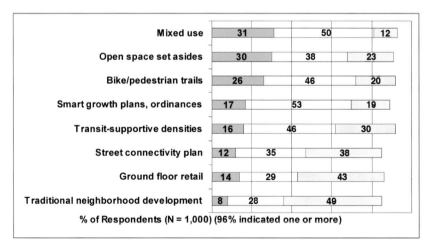

Figure 1-5. Smart growth reforms that promote walkability since 1993 in surveyed jurisdictions.

Focusing on elements found in walkable communities, respondents were askcd to indicate the specific measures their jurisdiction had implemented to support walking and physical activity. Since many codes are revised and reformed incrementally, respondents were asked whether the actions had been implemented to a large extent, to some extent, or not at all (Figure 1-5).

Mixed-use development was the most commonly implemented measure, with 31 percent indicating their jurisdiction permits it and an additional 50 percent having included such provisions to some extent (presumably they allowed it in some but not all districts). Also scoring high were bicycle and pedestrian trails, with 26 percent indicating they had required or encouraged the incorporation of such facilities into subdivisions since 1993, with an additional 46 percent having done so to some extent. Increasing development density near transit also scored high—16 percent indicated it had been implemented to a great extent, and 46 percent said it had been done to some extent. Perhaps the most broadly encouraging finding was the results for smart growth plans and policies. Seventeen percent indicated the jurisdiction had incorporated smart growth polices into plans, ordinances, and development review processes, and more than half (53 percent) said they had done so to some extent.

The Active Living Network

Many other nonprofit groups, advocacy, research organizations are also working on the active living initiatives. APA and other organizations are part of the Active Living Network, a consortium of organizations and an information clearinghouse created by the Robert Wood Johnson. On its website the Network is described as follows:

> [The Active Living Network] is a coordinated response to find creative approaches for integrating physical activity into American life. Rather than solely addressing obesity as an individual health problem, the Network focuses on how the built environment — including neighborhoods, transportation systems, buildings, parks and open space — can promote more active lives.
>
> To achieve this goal, the Active Living Network is building relationships among leaders in diverse professions such as urban planning, architecture, transportation planning, education, environment and public health. Together we work to identify opportunities for coordinated action and to promote activity-friendly environments in cities, schools, workplaces and neighborhoods.

RWJF also created three national program offices as part of the network. The program provided five-year grants to 25 communities across the U.S. to aid them in developing coordinated, interdisciplinary, public- and private-sector efforts to create an active community. Several of the grant recipient communities are highlighted in the case studies in this report. Active Living Research (ALR), based at San Diego State University, has provided six rounds of grants to interdisciplinary teams of researchers who are testing and evaluating the most effective built environment interventions to improve opportunities for physical activity. (In 2006, ALR expanded its mission to include research on nutritional issues related to obesity.) And finally, Active Living Leadership, which was initially based at San Diego State University but is now managed out of RWJF headquarters, provides grant support to several national organizations that represent elected and appointed officials at each level of government.

APA's charge was to focus directly on the input that planners can and should have on the issue and the tools and information planners will need to incorporate physical activity objectives into local planning processes.

A NEW PLANNING PARADIGM FOR ACTIVE COMMUNITIES: POINTS OF STRATEGIC INTERVENTION IN THE PLANNING PROCESS

Drawing on the expert opinion, planning, public health, and popular literature, and interactions with the numerous other organizations and entities researching, advocating, and implementing active community environments cited in the previous section, we set forth a conceptual framework to define the roles that planners have in modifying the built environment to encourage physical activity. The framework centers on what we have termed "the five strategic points of intervention" where planners can affect change:

1. Visioning and goal setting

2. Plans and planning

3. Implementation tools

4. Site design and development

5. Public facility siting

Underlying this framework is the growing body of evidence that supports the common sense beliefs held by many planners and health experts that the built environment has a direct effect on a person's ability, opportunity, and willingness to be physically active as part of their daily routine. That evidence has reached a level where we can now begin to put forward new planning and community design policies that will result in more active community environments.

Point 1. Visioning and Goal Setting

When citizens, planners, and stakeholder groups come together to prepare a new plan, the conversation typically begins with a discussion of shared values. Such groups brainstorm about how they would like their neighborhood, city, parks, or transportation system to look and to function.

Protecting and improving one's family's health and one's own health is a universally shared value. But in the thousands of jurisdictions, agencies, and other entities that prepare land-use plans, it is the exception for health and physical activity advocates or public health professionals to be present as stakeholders at visioning session. Their absence results in several missed opportunities. First, planners and public health practitioners could use such sessions to educate the public about how communities develop and the effect development patterns have on their ability to be physically active when following their daily routines.

Point 2. Plans and Planning

As described above, smart growth planning—a major focus of which is the creation of walkable, compact, mixed-use neighborhoods and a multimodal transportation network—are inherently supportive of increasing the physical activity of residents. In other words, smart growth has laid solid groundwork for planning to address health.

But it is important for health to be elevated to the level of other land-use and comprehensive plan goals (e.g., creating affordable housing, supporting economic development, and protecting open space) if jurisdictions are to be successful in creating active, healthy communities. Without direct involvement by health experts in the planning process, health has not been, nor is it likely to be, addressed in plans to any substantive degree. Creating opportunities for citizens to be physically active needs to be an explicit, not simply implied, goal in comprehensive plans, as well as many of the functional plans and plan elements that most jurisdictions prepare, including the transportation and circulation plan, bike and trails plan, housing plan, and parks and recreation plan, among others. It is not enough for planners and local officials to assume that, when implemented, a new bicycle and pedestrian plan will result in people becoming more active and healthier. Such plans need to document baseline health conditions and describe how

We have found "five strategic points of intervention" where planners can affect change.

It is not enough for planners and local officials to assume that, when implemented, a new bicycle and pedestrian plan will result in people becoming more active and healthier. Such plans need to document baseline health conditions and describe how such conditions will be addressed as the plan is implemented. They also need to prescribe how and when the effects of such change will be measured, monitored, and reported.

such conditions will be addressed as the plan is implemented. They also need to prescribe how and when the effects of such change will be measured, monitored, and reported.

Smart growth plans have also been touted as a potential solution to other health problems. For example, promoting compact, walkable developments and increasing transportation choices beyond the automobile can reduce car dependence for some families and thus improve air quality. A balanced plan for transportation would likely advocate or require narrower-than-typical streets as well as traffic calming in residential areas, which can reduce the incidence of motor vehicle/pedestrian accidents. Such accidents are the leading causes of death among persons 1 to 34 years old. Data from a 2005 preliminary report from the U.S. DOT's National Highway Traffic Safety Administration (NHTSA) indicated that 43,200 people died on U.S. highways in 2005, up from 42,636 in 2004.

On the environmental front, urban service limits or growth boundaries, which delineate the outermost points of an urbanized area to be served by sewer and water utilities, can help stem groundwater contamination by cutting down on the number of septic systems and redirecting future growth to areas already served by municipal utilities.

Figure 1-6. Factors determining transportation mode choice and physical activity level.

- Built environment factors
- Social/cultural factors
- Psychological, cognitive and emotional factors
- Attitudes and preferences
- Socioeconomic factors

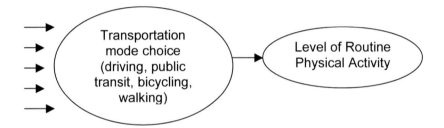

Point 3. Implementation Tools

Numerous modifications can be made to zoning and subdivision regulations to produce neighborhoods where residents have more opportunities to be active. First, jurisdictions can revise ordinances to permit mixed-use development where housing, shopping, and offices can coexist in the same building or in the same zoning districts. Going a step farther, zoning ordinances should be revised to include new urbanist or traditional neighborhood development (TND) provisions, either as an overlay district, as a requirement in certain districts, or communitywide. Such provisions, like other smart growth provisions, promote compact communities with services and principal locations within walking or biking distance.

Other tools include:

- increasing required development densities (i.e., the minimum number of dwelling units per acre);

- requiring sidewalks and/or trails in new developments and retrofitting already developed areas with sidewalks, trails, and bike paths, as well as instituting traffic calming measures (e.g., speed bumps, narrowing the drivers' field of vision; see Ewing 1999 and Hoyle 1995 for more detail);

- requiring new developments to include usable parks or open spaces that ideally connect to similar spaces in adjacent neighborhoods; and

- requiring street connectivity, where a grid or modified grid street network allows persons on foot, bike, or behind the wheel to travel from one neighborhood to another and one destination to another without having to depend on a crowded arterial street (see Handy et. al. 2003 for more detail).

In larger metropolitan areas, the provision of public transit and transit-oriented development (TOD) can add to residents' transportation choices.

Point 4. Site Design and Development

Factors of building design, site design, and the relationship of a building to its surroundings determine whether an area allows or promotes physical activity. These factors include the orientation of a building to the street, architectural details, building materials, windows, and sidewalks. For the most part, these elements are chosen or decided upon by the developer in concert with the planning agency, and, depending on their design, can either promote or prohibit pedestrian activity.

Many jurisdictions have also invested in new sidewalks, crosswalks, street lighting, public art, transit shelters, and street furniture to create pedestrian-oriented settings and public gathering places. Furthermore, zoning and planned unit development (PUD) regulations commonly contain provisions for developers to provide other amenities, such as landscaping, on-site pedestrian paths, awnings, and variety in building design. Such regulations often require that buildings be built right to the sidewalk rather than set back beyond surface parking and also require retail on the ground floor of multifamily residential and office buildings, multiple entrances for pedestrian convenience, and transparent windows on the first floor, all to create a lively street scene conducive to walking.

Ordinances can prohibit long, blank walls that deter people from walking by requiring large buildings to vary the blank wall by creating more inviting facades with windows, awnings, architectural features, and entrances. And finally, ordinances governing development in pedestrian-friendly areas now commonly allow developers to build less parking and to locate all or some of it on the side or rear of commercial buildings. The object is to minimize the amount of surface parking overall and to shape the public realm in a way that puts the people's safety and comfort ahead of the movement and accommodation of cars.

Point 5. Public Facility Siting

The location of public facilities and the design of the environments around them are keys to creating active communities. Unlike the other strategic points of intervention, planners tend to have much less influence over public facility siting and design. Instead, other local or federal government agencies with preemptive powers that override local plans and zoning rules make those decisions.

Post offices, schools, city hall, courthouses, and libraries serve as frequent destinations, popular community gathering places, and as visual, architectural focal points of a community. Post offices on Main Street provide a destination for residents interested in "purposeful" walking (i.e., getting some exercise while accomplishing errands at the same time). But in the last several decades, many such post offices in many small towns and suburbs have relocated to new, single-story processing facilities outside the city. Schools, in particular, as the sidebar notes, can serve as community centers.

The trend in the last several decades has been for school districts to build fewer and larger schools on sites disconnected from the places students live. At the same time, many smaller, older, neighborhood-based schools more likely to be accessible to kids on foot or by bike are shutting their doors. According to the CDC, in 2000 just 13 percent of school children walked to school, as compared to 1969, when 66 percent of kids walked to school (CDC 2002). According to parents, the two primary reasons why kids are driven rather than walk to school are, first, schools are too far for kids to walk, and

SCHOOLS AS CENTERS OF THE COMMUNITY

A 2003 report by the National Clearinghouse for Educational Facilities and other allied organizations addressed the critical backlog of school investment needs in the U.S. The report acknowledged that the pressing need to renovate, replace, and create many new schools presents a compelling opportunity to evaluate existing research about what constitutes an optimum learning environment. What they found was that all creative solutions, such as reducing school size, reconfiguring classrooms, and emphasizing lifelong and experiential learning, have one common theme: schools should be the centers of community. At their best, community-centered schools should:

• help meet a community's leisure, recreational, and wellness needs;

• be accessible to people of all ages;

• encourage more parental involvement in school activities; and

• contain shared public spaces that are accessible year round.

Community-centered schools are supportive of activity-friendly objectives. They would generally be smaller and located within neighborhoods, they could increase opportunities for kids to walk to school, and they would provide opportunities for all members of the community to use and enjoy recreational facilities and public spaces.

Source: National Clearinghouse for Educational Facilities 2003

second, the route they would have to walk is too dangerous (e.g., inadequate sidewalks, no crosswalks). At the high school level, the increasing rate of car ownership per household in recent decades means that kids are driving themselves to school in ever-growing numbers.

For younger children, the shift from a walk to a ride to school is, in part, prompted by changes in American family life. Households with two parents working full-time often lack the time to walk their children to school. Single working parents also opt to drive their kids to school rather than let them walk there unsupervised. Even kids that live within close proximity to their school are not walking or bicycling. The CDC has also found that 31 percent of kids that live within one mile of school walk or bike to school; in 1969, 90 percent did so (CDC 2002).

For mothers, the effect of serving as the family taxi driver is troubling. *High Mileage Moms*, a 1999 report by the Surface Transportation Policy Project, found that, on average, a typical mother travels 29 miles a day, taking five or more trips, spending more than an hour behind the wheel each day. That is 20 percent more driving than the amount of driving done by either single women or men, and constitutes time mothers could be spending with their family or getting exercise.

Clearly, more informed and thoughtful community planning and design and school board decisions about the location of schools is needed if we are to encourage parents and children to consider walking or biking to school as a viable option and as a means for children to get some necessary exercise.

CHAPTER 1 LIST OF REFERENCES

[This List of References is supplemented by a Master Resource List at the end of this PAS Report.]

CDC (Centers for Disease Control and Prevention). 2002. "Barriers to Children Walking and Biking to School – United States, 1999." *Journal of the American Medical Association* 288, no. 11 (September): 1,343–44.

_____. 1996. *Physical Activity and Health: A Report of the Surgeon General.* Atlanta, Ga.: CDC, National Center for Chronic Disease Prevention and Health Promotion.

Ewing, Reid. 1999. "Impacts of Traffic Calming." In *Urban Street Symposium: Conference Proceedings: Dallas, Texas, June 28-30, 1999.* Washington, D.C.: Transportation Research Board, 2000.

Frank, L.D., and P. Engelke. 2000. *How Land Use and Transportation Systems Impact Public Health: A Literature Review of the Relationship between Physical Activity and Built Form.* Atlanta, Ga.: Centers for Disease Control and Prevention, National Center for Chronic Disease Prevention and Health Promotion, Division of Nutrition and Physical Activity. www.cdc.gov/nccdphp/dnpa/pdf/aces-workingpaper1.pdf

Handy, Susan L., Robert G. Paterson, and Kent Butler. 2003. *Planning for Street Connectivity: Getting from Here to There.* Planning Advisory Service Report No. 515. Chicago: American Planning Association.

Hoyle, Cynthia. 1995. *Traffic Calming.* Planning Advisory Service Report No. 456. Chicago: American Planning Association.

CHAPTER 2

Defining Physical Activity and Active Living: Framing the Issue

By Rich Killingsworth

Since the dawn of human history, physical activity has played a primary role in good function, performance, and health. Only until the recent past century has physical activity been an often overlooked and somewhat confusing behavior. Overlooked because it appears that it has been or is about to be engineered out of daily routines. Confusing because most people have placed a variety of meanings and images to what was once a very simple behavior.

Physical activity is any movement of the skeletal muscles that results in energy expenditure (Caspersen et al. 1985). Physical activity in daily life can include occupational activity, sports, and household chores (Caspersen et al. 1985). The 1996 landmark report by the Surgeon General on Physical Activity and Health (U.S. Department of Health and Human Services 1996) recommends that everyone over the age of two years accumulate 30 minutes or more of moderately intense physical activity on most days of the week, further clarified to mean five or more days per week. Moderate activities include brisk walking, bicycling at about 10 m.p.h., mowing the lawn, heavy gardening, and many other activities. Alternatively, health benefits can be derived from participating in vigorous and strength-developing activities for at least 20 minutes on three or more days per week (ACSM 1995).

The following explanations will be helpful to clarify the differences between physical activity, exercise, physical fitness, and active living. Exercise is physical activity that is planned, structured, repetitive, and purposive in that improvement or maintenance of one or more of the components of physical fitness is an objective (Caspersen et al. 1985). Physical fitness is a set of attributes that are either health or skill related. The degree to which people have these attributes can be measured with specific tests related to speed, strength, flexibility, endurance, and several other attributes. Active living is a term recently added to the vocabulary of health promotion. Active living is a concept that has emerged from a growing movement that suggests the built environment, especially transportation choice, affects decisions to be physically active. Active living has been defined as a way of life that integrates physical activity into daily routines. In essence, this term addresses the opportunity to identify activities such as walking or biking to destinations, taking the stairs instead of the elevator, or pushing a lawn mower instead or riding it as ways to integrate physical activity in one's lifestyle. While these behaviors are specifically utilitarian, the concept of active living also stretches into the issue of altering one's lifestyle to merely be more active and to be more active throughout the course of the day.

These definitions are helpful in that they clarify the primary goal to improve health is to increase physical activity or simply to get people moving enough to achieve the recommended dose of activity.

WHAT ARE THE BENEFITS OF PHYSICAL ACTIVITY?

Regular physical activity increases cardiovascular functional capacity and decreases myocardial oxygen demand at any level, in healthy people as well as those with cardiovascular disease. In order to maintain these benefits, regular physical activity is required (Fletcher et al. 1996).

Physical activity has been associated with lower risk of hip fracture, coronary events, and total cardiovascular effects in older women and decreased cardiovascular disease in older men. The Nurse's Health Study, which followed 61,200 postmenopausal women for 12 years, found that active women had a 55 percent lower risk of hip fracture than sedentary women (Feskanich et al. 2002). Among women who did no other exercise, walking for at least four hours per week was associated with a 41 percent lower risk of hip fracture than women who walked less than one hour per week (Feskanich et al. 2002). Both walking and vigorous activity have been associated with substantial reductions in the incidence of cardiovascular events in postmenopausal women (Manson et al. 2002). An increasing physical activity score had a strong, graded, inverse association with the risk of both coronary events and total cardiovascular events (Manson et al. 2002). Women who walked or exercised briskly at least 2.5 hours per week showed a 30 percent risk reduction in cardiovascular disease, whereas time spent sitting increased risk (Manson et al. 2002). These findings were true in

Active living is a concept that has emerged from a growing movement that suggests the built environment, especially transportation choice, affects decisions to be physically active.

Caucasian and African-American women, across ages, groups, and categories of body mass index (Manson et al. 2002).

In a study that examined men ages 40-59 and then followed up 20 years later, physical activity was inversely associated with several hemostatic and inflammatory variables. All currently active men, regardless of their activity levels 20 years prior, showed lower levels of these variables than currently inactive men (Wannamethee et al. 2002). The benefit of physical activity on cardiovascular disease may be at least partly a result of a short-term effect through these mechanisms (Wannamethee et al. 2002).

Scientific evidence is beginning to accumulate that physical activity is a form of primary prevention for cancer (Friedenreich and Orenstein 2002). After adjusting for age, smoking status, body mass index, alcohol intake and social class, the risk of total cancers was significantly reduced in men reporting moderately vigorous and vigorous activity. No health benefits were seen for less than vigorous activity (Wannamethee et al. 2001). More research is needed to discover the mechanisms involved and to explore the link between physical activity and risk of cancer for subsets of the population (Friedenreich and Orenstein 2002).

WHAT ARE THE RISKS OF INACTIVITY?

A sedentary lifestyle has been linked to several morbidity outcomes (U. S. Deartment of Health and Human Services 1996). Adults with chronic disease who were physically inactive had higher observed mortality rates than those who were physically active, in a three-year follow-up study (Martinson et al. 2001). Research has shown that light to moderate activity led to lowered risk of overweight for men (Ching et al. 1996). Ching (1996) also identifies a strong correlation with diabetes. The common element in patients who develop adolescent-onset Type 2 Diabetes is extreme obesity, compounded by family obesity, high fat diet, and sedentary lifestyle (Pinhas-Hamiel et al. 2000).

The National Longitudinal Study of Adolescent Health also found that for boys, the odds of overweight are nearly 50 percent higher with high levels of TV viewing (Gordon-Larsen 2002). Television watching may lead to higher caloric intake, which may result in the relationship between television viewing and being overweight (Robinson 2001). Among Caucasian boys, the odds of being overweight decreased with high levels of moderate to vigorous physical activity (Gordon-Larsen 2002). Ethnic differences in results may be a result of the complex interaction between socioeconomic, environmental, and cultural influences (Gordon-Larsen 2002).

Being overweight in adolescence is particularly detrimental to later health outcomes. Data from the Third Harvard Growth Study was used to follow up with 309 subjects in 1988 when they reached mid-life (Must et al. 1992). Being overweight in adolescence predicted a broad range of adverse health effects that were independent of adult weight after 55 years of follow-up (Must et al. 1992). Being overweight in adolescence was associated with increased risk of all-cause mortality and disease-specific mortality among men. Men and women classified as overweight in adolescence had increased risk of morbidity from coronary heart disease and artherosclerosis (Must et al. 1992).

Trends in cardiovascular risk factors were studied in 25-74 year olds, based on four surveys done in Minneapolis, St. Paul, between 1980 and 1982 and 1995-1997 (Arnett et al. 2002). Body mass index increased substantially across the four surveys and the proportion of the population that is not regularly exercising increased between 1990-1992 and 1995-1997 (Arnett et al. 2002). Between 1980 and 1997, unfavorable trends in total cholesterol levels, hypercholesterolemia, adiposity, and physical activity were paralleled by positive changes like decreasing fat consumption, smoking, and hypertension (Arnett et al. 2002).

Economic calculations suggest that increasing regular, moderate physical activity levels among the 88 million inactive adults over the age of 15 would have reduced annual U.S. medical costs by $76.6 billion in 2000 (Pratt et al. 2000).

THE CONNECTION TO OBESITY

Obesity is defined as having a body mass index (Kg/m^2) greater than or equal to 30 (www.cdc.gov, accessed on September 11, 2003). Results from the 2003-2004 National Health and Nutrition Examination Survey (NHANES), using measured heights and weights, indicate that an estimated 66 percent of U.S. adults are either overweight or obese (NCEH 2006). (See Figure 2-1.) One of the national health objectives for 2010 is to reduce the prevalence of obesity among adults to less than 15 percent. However, the NHANES 2003-2004 data for persons age 20 years and over suggest an increase in the proportion of obese adults in the U.S., where the estimated age-adjusted prevalence moved upward from a previous level of 23 percent in NHANES III (which measured obesity in the period 1988-1994) to a new level of approximately 32 percent.

FIGURE 2-1. OBESITY TRENDS* AMONG U.S. ADULTS

(*BMI ≥30, or about 30 lbs overweight for 5' 4" person)

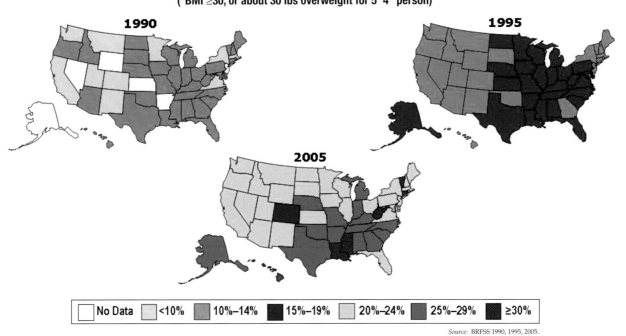

Source: BRFSS 1990, 1995, 2005.

Prevalence of overweight among youth in the U.S. ranges from 11-24 percent (Troiano and Flegal 1999). Generally, 85th-95th percentile is the definition of obesity (Troiano and Flegal 1999). Percentiles are based on a variety of anthropometric measures. Despite varying results, many studies confirm that overweight prevalence among youth has increased dramatically (Troiano and Flegal 1999). The lack of a general increase in energy intake among youth between 1970s and 1990s suggests that physical inactivity is the major cause of increased overweight (Troiano et al. 2000). Overweight youths tend to consume a greater number of their calories from beverages than their peers (Troiano et al. 2000). This public health problem must be addressed through primary prevention methods such as increasing physical activity among young people and decreasing the consumption of nonnutritive foods and beverages (Troiano et al. 2000, Troiano et al. 1995). There is also evidence that food advertisements lead to food preferences in children (Wadden et al. 2002). In addition to improving resources available for physical activity, healthy food choices should replace fast foods and soft drinks in schools (Wadden et al. 2002).

The prevalence of obesity-related comorbidities, including cardiovascular disease and diabetes, emphasizes the need for greater efforts to prevent and treat obesity rather than simply treating its comorbidities (Must et al. 1999).

BARRIERS TO PHYSICAL ACTIVITY

According to the 2002 Behavioral Risk Factor Surveillance System of the Centers for Disease Control and Prevention, 24.4 percent of Americans are physically inactive (accessed from www.cdc.gov, October 10, 2003). Inactivity tends to be the highest among Americans 65+ years of age, women, racial/ethnic minorities, people with fewer than 12 years of education, and those with a household income of less than $20,000 (Weinstein et al. 1999). The association between low perceived neighborhood safety and self-reported levels of physical inactivity were found only in older adults (Weinstein et al. 1999). For women, lack of hills in one's neighborhood, absence of enjoyable scenery and infrequently seeing others' exercising have also been linked to inactivity (King et al. 2000).

Women living in rural areas in the southern U.S. have been found to be more sedentary than urban women (Wilcox et al. 2000). Rural women reported more personal barriers to leisure-time physical activity and greater body mass indices than urban women (Wilcox et al. 2000). Rural women have been less likely than urban women to report the presence of sidewalks, streetlights, and high crime in their neighborhoods. Rural women are also less likely to report access to exercise facilities and seeing others exercising in their neighborhoods (Wilcox et al. 2000). Urban women reported that their top three barriers to physical activity were, in order, lack of time, lack of energy, and being too tired. Rural women reported the top barriers as caregiving duties, lack of time, and lack of energy (Wilcox et al. 2000).

According to the Third National Health and Nutrition Examination Survey, conducted by the National Center for Health Statistics, for all race/ethnic groups, persons living below the poverty line reported more leisure-time inactivity than persons living above the poverty line (Crespo et al. 2000). Across education levels, minority men and women were more inactive in their leisure time than Caucasians. Further research should examine the effects of acculturation, safety, social support, and environmental factors in increasing physical activity among minority groups (Crespo et al., 2000). The personal and social motivations for activity, as well as lifestyle and environmental factors, must be explored further (Sherwood and Jeffery 2000).

In a study of older Americans, the most significant predictor of leisure-time activity was the leisure-time physical activity of one's spouse (Sternfeld et al. 2002). This was true for all couples except those who engage in less than brisk physical activity. Of the 2,073 participants surveyed, women who lived with others (not a spouse or independently) were more likely to engage in less-than-brisk activity (Sternfeld et al. 2002). Men with fewer than six social contacts were only half as likely as those with more contacts to engage in moderate or highly vigorous activities (Sternfeld et al. 2002).

More than 15,000 Europeans were asked about the most important barriers to increasing physical activity. Twenty-eight percent stated that work and study commitments were prohibitive and 25 percent said they didn't believe they were the 'sporty type' (Zunft 1999). Eighteen percent of women felt that caring for children and/or elderly relatives was an important barrier to physical activity (Zunft 1999). The most important reasons for Europeans to be physically active were: to maintain good health (42 percent), release tension (30 percent),

According to the 2002 Behavioral Risk Factor Surveillance System of the Centers for Disease Control and Prevention, 24.4 percent of Americans are physically inactive.

and get fit (30 percent) (Zunft 1999). Those aged 55+ years said that "good health" was their primary motivation for physical activity (Zunft 1999).

INTERVENTIONS TO PROMOTE PHYSICAL ACTIVITY

The current epidemic of obesity is caused largely by an environment that promotes excessive food and beverage consumption and discourages physical activity (French et al. 2001). The number of fast-food restaurants increased 147 percent between 1972 and 1995 (French et al. 2001). Sedentary behavior is linked to increased television viewing and reliance on automobiles for transportation (French et al. 2001). In order to improve the health of the public, we must support walking and bicycling, post signs to promote stair usage, and redesign neighborhoods to encourage physical activity (French et al. 2001). Many interventions have focused on changing individual behavior, yet policy and environmental approaches can have a greater impact because they influence the whole culture over a longer period of time (King et al. 1995). Passive approaches must be promoted, such as restricting downtown centers to walking and biking only, making stairways more safe and convenient, and developing mixed-use areas (King et al. 1995).

LESSONS LEARNED: PROMOTING PHYSICAL ACTIVITY AT THE LOCAL LEVEL

In 2002, the Robert Wood Johnson Foundation awarded 25 communities funding to development projects that would promote walking, biking, and other forms of physical activity. A 2006 report by the Foundation that is based upon interviews of key representatives from each of the 25 communities drew the following 12 general lessons about what worked and what did not.

- Building the community's capacity to implement change is important, not only to the initial success of a project but also to sustaining behavioral change.
- Communities value opportunities to learn from other communities.
- A local champion to spearhead an initiative and encourage community investment can be extremely helpful.
- Mayors, in particular, can be key levers of change in a community. They are often able to garner the resources to sustain change.
- Programs to provide social support for physical activity in community settings need staff and are best housed in stable institutions able to support ongoing personnel costs.
- To ensure use, paths, trails, and parks need to be promoted and maintained, and that requires community sponsors and long-term partnerships.
- To engage lower-income and minority residents in physical activity, programming should be adapted to their circumstances and needs.
- Making physical activity fun, social, and not intimidating is beneficial, especially when trying to reach the least active.
- Over time, a walking program may spur development of broader programming to meet a variety of needs and preferences.
- Pedometers can motivate new walkers but need oversight for optimal use.
- Without significant funding and support, service organizations that sponsor physical activity programs can find it challenging to take on additional activities, such as research and evaluation.
- Messages promoting physical activity must be intense if they are to compete successfully with other messages and influences.

Source: Heroux. 2005

An evaluation of the effectiveness of various approaches in increasing physical activity was done, using behavior change and increased aerobic capacity as the measures of success (Kahn et al. 2002). Two informational interventions were effective, both point-of-decision prompts to encourage stair usage and communitywide physical activity campaigns (Kahn et al. 2002). Three behavioral and social interventions were effective, school-based physical education, social support in community settings, and individually adapted behavior change. One environmental intervention was effective, enhancing access to places for physical activity in combination with informational support (Kahn et al. 2002). The key mediators hypothesized to influence behavioral outcomes for adults and youth are: behavioral and cognitive processes of change, self-efficacy, decisional balance, social support, and enjoyment (Lewis et al. 2002).

Community-level indicators (CLIs) based on observations of aspects of the community may supplement individual measures in evaluating community-based programs (Cheadle et al. 2000). The Centers for Disease Control and Prevention issued a list of indicators grouped into four categories, policy and regulation, information, environmental change, and behavioral outcome (Cheadle et al. 2000). CLIs may be less expensive to collect than individual measures since they are unobtrusive and non-reactive (Cheadle et al. 2000). They are also derived from the community environment, which is a target of many interventions (Cheadle et al. 2000).

Most public health issues are best addressed through a combination of active and passive strategies (Schmid et al. 1995). The 50 percent reduction in motor vehicle fatality rates per mile driven over the past decades is a result of improved roadways, automobiles, speed limits, seat belt usage campaigns, drunk driving legislation, law enforcement, driver education and safer driving (Schmid et al. 1995). As health agencies move away from direct service to empowering communities to address underlying public health problems, they must ensure that policy and environmental options are included in public discourse (Schmid et al. 1995). Tax breaks for cafeterias that offer healthy choices, policies that require subdivisions to include sidewalks, and school facilities open to the public after school hours may be seen as radical today but will one day be considered common and necessary to ensure public health (Schmid et al. 1995).

While physical activity is a complex behavior, a study by Paffenbarger (1993) suggests that it is never too late to obtain the health benefits of participating in physical activity.

IT'S NEVER TOO LATE

While physical activity is a complex behavior, a study by Paffenbarger (1993) suggests that it is never too late to obtain the health benefits of participating in physical activity. Subjects in the study who began participating in physical activity after years of inactivity had reduced mortality rates when compared to those who remained sedentary. This benefit was apparent even for the men who became physically active after the age of 60. This conclusion provides an opportunity for public health practitioners to promote moderate physical activity across all age segments.

Another opportunity is to highlight the main function of physical activity—to get people moving and increasing physical activity throughout the day through various options such a utilitarian, recreational, occupational, and household. The most opportunistic recommendation seems to be encouraging people to walk or bike instead of driving whenever possible. Once the initial goal of moving more has been accomplished and sustained, this may provide an orientation to participate in other physical activities that may include exercise options. The public health goal is to shift enough people to achieve the recommended does of physical activity (30 minutes of moderately intense activity on at least five days per week) to seek a demonstrable difference in public health outcomes related to inactivity (obesity, diabetes, hypertension, etc.).

The closing message regarding physical activity is that the literature provides substantial evidence that it is a key behavior to promote better health outcomes among all people and throughout the lifespan. The evidence also suggests that city planners, transportation engineers, urban designers, landscape architects, developers, and others can play a significant role in how we promote physical activity through the built environment. If we expect to achieve the goal of having neighborhoods, towns, cities, and regions promote the health of their residents, we need to consider more carefully how decisions related to the built environment can impact the choice to be physically active and healthier.

CHAPTER 2 LIST OF REFERENCES

[*This List of References is supplemented by a Master Resource List at the end of the PAS Report.*]

ACSM (American College of Sports Medicine), and U.S. Centers for Disease Control and Prevention. 1993. "Summary Statement: Workshop on physical activity and public health." *Sports Medicine Bulletin* 28 (4): 7.

Arnett, Donna K., Paul G. McGovern, David R. Jacobs, Jr., et al. 2002. "Fifteen-Year Trends in Cardiovascular Risk Factors (1980–1982 through 1995–1997)." *American Journal of Epidemiology* 156: 929–35.

Caspersen, C. J., K.E. Powell, and G.M. Christenson. 1985. "Physical Activity, Exercise, and Physical Fitness: Definitions and Distinctions for Health-Related Research." *Public Health Reports* 100 (2): 126-31.

Cheadle, C., T.D. Sterling, et al. 2000. "Promising Community-Level Indicators for Evaluating Cardiovascular Health-Promotion Programs." *Health Education Research* 15, no. 1: 109–16.

Ching, P. L., W. C. Willett, E. B. Rimm, et al. 1996. "Activity Level and Risk of Overweight in Male Health Professionals." *American Journal of Public Health* 86, no. 1: 25–30.

Crespo, C. J., E. Smit, R. E. Andersen, et al. 2000. "Race/Ethnicity, Social Class and Their Relation to Physical Inactivity During Leisure Time: Results From the Third National Health and Nutrition Examination Survey, 1988–1994." *American Journal of Preventive Medicine* 18, no. 1: 46–53.

Feskanich, Diane, Walter Willett, and Graham Colditz. 2002. "Walking and Leisure-Time Activity and Risk of Hip Fracture in Postmenopausal Women." *Journal of the American Medical Association* 288: 2,300-06.

Fletcher, Gerald F., et al. 1996. "Statement On Exercise: Benefits And Recommendations For Physical Activity Programs For All Americans." *Circulation* 94, no. 4: 857–62.

French, Simone A., Mary Story, and Robert W. Jeffery. 2001. "Environmental Influences on Eating and Physical Activity." *Annual Review of Public Health.* 22:309–35.

Friedenreich, C., and M. Orenstein. 2002. "Physical Activity and Cancer Prevention: Etiologic Evidence and Biological Mechanisms." *Journal of Nutrition.* 132: 3456S-64S.

Gordon-Larsen, P., L. S. Adair, and B.M. Popkin. 2002a. "U.S. Adolescent Physical Activity and Inactivity Patterns Are Associated with Overweight: The National Longitudinal Study of Adolescent Health." *Obesity Research* 10: 141–49.

_____. 2002b. "Ethnic Differences in Physical Activity and Inactivity Patterns and Overweight Status." *Obesity Research* 10, no. 3: 141–49.

Heroux, Janet. 2005. *Lessons Learned: Promoting Physical Activity at the Local Level.* A Grant Results Special Report. Princeton, N.J.: The Robert Wood Johnson Foundation.

Kahn, E. B., L. T. Ramsey, R. C. Brownson, et al. 2002. "The Effectiveness of Interventions to Increase Physical Activity: A Systematic Review." *American Journal of Preventive Medicine* 22, no. 4: 73–107.

King, A. C., C. Castro, S. Wilcox, et al. 2000. "Personal and Environmental Factors Associated with Physical Inactivity Among Different Racial-Ethnic Groups of U.S. Middle-Aged and Older-Aged Women." *Health Psychology* 19 (July): 354–64.

King, A. C., R. W. Jeffery, F. Fridinger, et al. 1995. "Environmental and Policy Approaches to Cardiovascular Disease Prevention through Physical Activity: Issues and Opportunities." *Health Education Quarterly.* November 22, no. 4: 499–511.

Lewis, B. A., B. H. Marcus, R. R. Pate, and A. L. Dunn. 2002. "Psychosocial Mediators of Physical Activity Behavior Among Adults and Children." *American Journal of Preventive Medicine* 23, no. 2: 26–35.

Manson, JoAnn E., Philip Greenland, Andrea Z. LaCroix, et al. 2002. "Walking Compared with Vigorous Exercise for the Prevention of Cardiovascular Events in Women." *The New England Journal of Medicine* 347 (September): 716–25.

Martinson, Brian C., Patrick J. O'Connor, and Nicolaas P. Pronk. 2001. "Physical Inactivity and Short-term All-Cause Mortality in Adults With Chronic Disease." *Archives of Internal Medicine* 161 (May)): 1,173–80.

Must, Aviva, Jennifer Spadano, Eugenie H. Coakley, et al. 1999. "The Disease Burden Associated With Overweight and Obesity." *Journal of the American Medical Association* 282 (October): 1,523–29.

Must, A, P. F. Jacques, G. E. Dallal, C. J. Bajema, and W. H. Dietz. 1992. "Long Term Morbidity and Mortality of Overweight Adolescents: A Follow-Up of the Harvard Growth Study of 1922 to 1935." *New England Journal of Medicine* 327: 1,350–55.

NCEH (National Center for Environmental Health); Centers for Disease Control and Prevention. 2006. "Prevalence of Overweight and Obesity Among Adults: United States, 2003-2004." www.cdc.gov/nchs/products/pubs/pubd/hestats/obese03_04/overwght_adult_03.htm.

Paffenbarger, R.S., R.T. Hyde et al. 1993. "The Association of Changes in Physical-activity Level and other Lifestyle Characteristics with Mortality Among Men." *New England Journal of Medicine* 328, no. 8: 538–45.

Pate, R. R., M. Pratt, M. Blair, et al. 1995. "Physical Activity and Public Health: A Recommendation from the Centers for Disease Control and Prevention and the American College of Sports Medicine." *Journal of American Medical Association* 273, no. 5: 402–07.

Pinhas-Hamiel, O. and P. Zeitler. 2000. "Who is the Wise Man? The One Who Foresees Consequences: Childhood Obesity, New Associated Comorbidity and Prevention." *Preventive Medicine* 31 (December): 702–05.

Pratt, M., C. A. Macera, and G. Wang. 2000. "Higher Direct Medical Costs Associated With Physical Inactivity." *Physician and Sportsmedicine* 28, no. 10: 63–70.

Robinson, T.N. 2002. "Television Viewing and Childhood Obesity." *Pediatric Clinics of North America* 48, no. 4: 1,017–25.

Schmid, T. L., M. Pratt, and E. Howze. 1995. "Policy as Intervention: Environmental and Policy Approaches to the Prevention of Cardiovascular Disease." *American Journal of Public Health* 85, no. 9: 1,207–11.

Sherwood, Nancy E. and Robert W. Jeffery. 2000. "The Behavioral Determinants of Exercise: Implications for Physical Activity Interventions." *Annual Review of Nutrition* 20 (July): 21–44.

Stein, Cynthia J. and Graham A. Colditz. "The Epidemic of Obesity." *Journal of Clinical Endocrinology and Metabolism* 89, no. 6: 2,522–25.

Sternfeld, Barbara, Long Ngo, William A. Satariano, and Ira B. Tager. 2002. "Associations of Body Composition with Physical Performance and Self-reported Functional Limitation in Elderly Men and Women." *American Journal of Epidemiology* 156: 110–21.

Troiano, R. P., K. M. Flegal, and R. J. Kuczmarski, et al. 1995. "Overweight Prevalence and Trends for Children and Adolescents. The National Health and Nutrition Examination Surveys, 1963 to 1991." *Archives of Pediatric and Adolescent Medicine* 149, no. 10.

Troiano, R.P. and K. M. Flegal. 1999. "Overweight Prevalence Among Youth in the United States: Why So Many Different Numbers?" *International Journal of Obesity* 23 (March): s22–s27. Supplement.

Troiano, R. P., R. R. Briefel, M. D. Carroll, and K. Bialostosky. 2000. "Energy and Fat Intakes of Children and Adolescents in the United States: Data from the National Health and Nutrition Examination Surveys." *The American Journal of Clinical Nutrition* 72, no. 5: 1,343s–53s. Supplement.

U. S. Department of Health and Human Services. 1996. *Physical Activity and Health: A Report of the Surgeon General.* Atlanta, Ga.: U.S. Department of Health and Human Services, Centers for Disease Control and Prevention, National Center for Chronic Disease Prevention and Health Promotion.

Wadden, TA, K. D. Brownell, and G. D. Foster. 2002. "Obesity: Responding to the Global Epidemic." *Journal of Consulting and Clinical Psychology* 70: 510–25.

Wannamethee, S. G., A. G. Shaper, and M. Walker. 2001. "Physical Activity and Risk of Cancer in Middle-Aged Men." *British Journal of Cancer* 85, no. 9: 1,311–16.

Wannamethee, S. Goya, D. Gordon, O. Lowe et al. 2002. "Physical Activity and Hemostatic and Inflammatory Variables in Elderly Men." *Circulation* 105: 1,785.

Weinstein, A., P. Feiglcy, P. Pullen, L. Mann, and L. Redman. 1999. "Neighborhood Safety and the Prevalence of Physical Activity—Selected States, 1996." *MMWR: Morbidity and Mortality Weekly Reports* 48: 143–46.

Wilcox, Sara, Cynthia Castro, Abby C. King, et al. 2000. "Determinants of Leisure Time Physical Activity in Rural Compared with Urban Older and Ethnically Diverse Women in the United States." *Journal of Epidemiology and Community Health* 54 (September): 667–72.

Zunft, H.J., and D. Friebe. 1999. "Perceived Benefits and Barriers to Physical Activity in a Nationally Representative Sample in the European Union." *Public Health Nutrition* 2 (March): 153–60.

CHAPTER 3

Reconnecting with Our Roots:
A Critical History of American Planning and
Public Health for the Twenty-First Century

By Jason Corburn

The emergence of urban planning as a profession and academic discipline had its basis in nineteenth century public health initiatives, including tenement housing reforms, the construction of urban water supply and sewerage systems, and the design of parks and playgrounds. The common origins of the urban planning and public health professions are also rooted in a view of the city as pathogenic and disorderly, requiring interventions to make urban areas more "regular and disciplined." While having similar visions of the city, the work of American professionals in each field diverged throughout the twentieth century, contributing to health disparities between urban and suburban populations and a failure to recognize the connections between, for example, land-use decisions and public health. I will show that the challenges facing the reconnection of the fields today are a direct, determined consequence of each field's history, and that if we do not wish to repeat past mistakes, we should learn lessons from the past to guide us into the future.

Urban design strategies to increasing physical activity and reducing obesity tend to ignore issues of political power, governance, institutional design, and epistemology that can influence whether interventions address the root causes of poor health, namely poverty, discrimination, and inequality more generally,

This chapter offers a critical historical analysis of the connections and disconnects between the fields of planning and public health from the latter half of the nineteenth through the twentieth century and offers some lessons for reconnecting the fields in the twenty-first century. While much of the recent work calling for reintegrating planning and public health has focused on specific urban design strategies that might, for instance, increase physical activity and reduce obesity, this chapter suggests that these approaches tend to ignore issues of political power, governance, institutional design, and epistemology that can influence whether interventions address the root causes of poor health, namely poverty, discrimination, and inequality more generally (Dannenberg et al. 2003; Fox et al. 2003; Frumkin 2002; Killingsworth et al. 2003; RWJF 2004).

This chapter seeks to extend the current discourse on reconnecting planning and public health by offering a synthesis of two vast and complex fields using secondary sources and drawing lessons for planning theory and practice today. I highlight persistent tendencies that emerge from critical events and movements within each field, ultimately revealing that both American public health and urban planning adopted four interrelated political themes.

1. Each field responds to real or perceived urban health crises through *physical removal and displacement*—of wastes, infrastructure, and people—primarily immigrants and African-Americans. This is evident from the waste removal programs of the sanitary era through the discriminatory housing and urban renewal policies of the post-War period.

2. *Scientific rationality* along with economic efficiency arguments act as the justification for most urban health interventions. Restoring order and normalcy to "pathogenic" cities with scientific methods and tools of neoliberal economics, not a vision of the healthy city, is the driving paradigm in both fields.

3. A third theme is the belief in *moral environmentalism*, or that rational physical and urban designs can change social conditions, particularly for the poor.

4. Finally, the *increasing professionalization* in each field disconnected the once common knowledge base and practices of planning and public health. Professionalization also helped create specialized bureaucracies, issue "silos," and an elite corps of technocrats with distinct disciplinary training, further disconnecting the fields.

To be explicit, by public health I am referring to public policies, practices, and processes that influence the distribution of disease, death, and well being for populations, or what the field generally calls health promotion. I use the Institute of Medicine (1988, 7) definition of public health. IOM defines its mission as:

> fulfilling society's interest in assuring the conditions in which people can be healthy....[T]he committee defines the substance of public health as: organized community efforts aimed at the prevention of disease and promotion of health. It links many disciplines and rests upon the scientific core of epidemiology.... [T]he committee defines the organizational framework of public health to encompass both activities undertaken within the formal structure of government and the associated efforts of private and voluntary organizations and individuals.

When using the term planning, I am describing public policies, practices and processes that influence both urban populations and the built environment of the city. I conceive planning as much more than land use and design, but also as the organizing of information, forecasting and modeling complex systems, and structuring public processes that can include or exclude impacted populations.

1850s–1900: MIASMA AND THE SANITARY CITY

On the eve of the Civil War, American cities were rapidly industrializing and trying to cope with overcrowded housing, noxious industrial, human, and animal wastes, and devastating outbreaks of infectious diseases. Characterized as dark and dirty slums, urban neighborhoods were blamed for the social "pathologies" of urban life, including violence, crime, "loose morals, bad habits, intemperance and idleness" (Boyer 1983, 17). Newly established municipal sanitary commissions in America adopted a utilitarian approach for justifying interventions (Duffy 1990) and, as Burrows and Wallace (1999, 785) note, made appeals for decent housing "not just as a measure of humanity, of justice to the poor, but as a matter of self interest. Bad housing meant sick workers, and sick workers meant lower profits, higher relief outlays, and higher taxes." Sanitary engineers also built new urban infrastructure, such as street-beds, freshwater and sewage systems, and filled in marsh and coastal wetlands where disease was thought to breed (Melosi 2000). New building codes specified design guidelines to improve conditions inside buildings, such as ventilation, light, and water closet design, but similar codes were not passed specifying design guidelines for the healthy neighborhood (Peterson 1979). Sanitarians tended to address health issues by employing emerging technologies to remove waste by, for instance, piping it away from cities into rivers and oceans, burning it and using the ash for land filling, or dumping it into "waste" marsh lands (Tarr 1996). Technology also improved living conditions, as the advent of the electric street car helped eliminate the stench and filth from manure and stables.

On the eve of the Civil War, American cities were rapidly industrializing and trying to cope with overcrowded housing, noxious industrial, human, and animal wastes, and devastating outbreaks of infectious diseases.

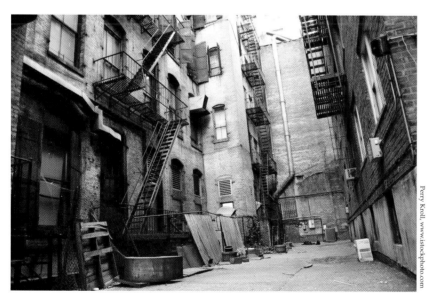

Perry Kroll, www.istockphoto.com

New York City developed the first citywide zoning code in 1916 in an effort to protect the public health and private property values. The spread of infectious disease among immigrant populations living in overcrowded tenements, such as the one shown here on the Lower East Side of Manhattan, was a major impetus for the city to enact the code.

The tendencies of sanitary engineers to remove waste had three displacement effects that would continue to characterize planning and public health throughout the twentieth century. First, by emphasizing waste removal and not reduction in the consumption patterns that created waste, sanitarians help institutionalize the idea that the "solution to pollution was dilution" (Melosi 1973). Ecosystems became the sinks for urban pollution. Second, sanitarians shifted the responsibility for waste from private industry and individuals to the state (Tarr 1996). Finally, by emphasizing engineered interventions, sanitarians advanced the idea that social, political, and economic problems could be best addressed through advances in science and technology.

When removing the miasma didn't seem to reduce disease, the sick were removed from society. *Contagion*, the belief in the direct passage of poison from one person to another led to large quarantines of immigrants and justified state-sponsored interventions in the economy, such as controlling shipping (Markel 1997). By 1893 the National Quarantine Act was passed, mandating that the Marine Hospital Service (later renamed the United States Public Health Service) screen foreigners at state quarantine stations and prevent the admission of "idiots, insane persons, . . . persons likely to become a public charge [and] persons suffering from a loathsome or dangerous contagious disease" (Mullan 1989, 41).

There are a number of examples during this era of state-sponsored quarantines targeted at immigrants. In 1892, the Port Authority of New York quarantined all passengers aboard ships arriving from Southern and Eastern Europe where a cholera outbreak had occurred. By 1900, Chinese immigrants were regularly detained at Angel Island and interrogated for diseases such as bubonic plague. In 1916, during an epidemic of poliomyletis, New York City's Department of Health began forcibly separating children from their parents and placing them in quarantine. However, wealthy parents were allowed to keep their stricken children at home if they could provide a separate room and medical care for their child (Rosen 1993).

Practices during this era that linked planning and public health included the sanitary survey, park and playground planning, and the work of settlement houses. After a devastating yellow fever outbreak in and around Memphis in 1878, a sanitary survey was launched to describe every street, structure, and individual lot within the city to determine the environmental conditions that might "breed" diseases (Peterson 1979, 90). Employing physicians, chemists, engineers, and others, the Memphis survey canvassed neighborhoods house-by-house and block-by-block, eventually recommending a comprehensive, citywide approach for guiding planning, including building a new water supply and sewer system, destroying shanties, damming bayous, developing a park along the shoreline, and repaving streets (Duffy 1990, 134).

While planning and public health both addressed sanitation and housing reforms during this time, the driving ideology was physical removal, of both "environmental miasmas" and "undesirable and sick" people.

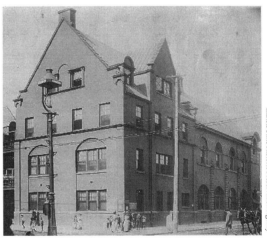

Hull House in Chicago played an important part in the Settlement House Movement of the late nineteenth century. The movement sought to house and to feed poor and working class immigrants, and to provide social and educational opportunities at the neighborhood level.

Illinois State Historic Preservation Agency

Planners in this era also sought to alleviate the crowded living conditions in cities by constructing "breathing spaces," such as parks and outdoor recreation areas. The playground movement challenged the idea that urban parks should only be places of leisure and contemplation and advocated for recreation spaces, especially for children. The movement, organized largely by women, advocated for urban play spaces next to schools so that gymnasiums, reading rooms, and baths could all be used for children's recreation, literacy, and hygiene.

Public baths were another sanitarian approach to removing moral and physical miasma. A private charity, the New York Association for Improving the Condition of the Poor, is credited with building one of the first public baths for the poor, driven largely by the belief that slum dwellers needed to be cleansed of moral failures and physical dirt (Duffy 1990).

Reformers in the Settlement House Movement organized and educated new immigrants while also providing impoverished neighborhood residents with food, day care, bathing facilities, libraries, art, and social events (Lubove 1974). The women of Hull House in Chicago, influenced by the burgeoning Chicago School of Sociology that initiated the study of the neighborhood effects on well-being, worked with residents to document unsanitary neighborhood and workplace conditions and advocated on behalf of residents for new social policies (Hull House Residents 1970). It must be noted, however, that, while the Settlement House movement embraced immigrants, it often refused to serve impoverished African-Americans.

By the end of the nineteenth century, modern American urban planning emerged as a field that used physical interventions to respond to urban public health crises. While planning and public health both addressed sanitation and housing reforms during this time, the driving ideology was physical removal, of both "environmental miasmas"— garbage, waste water, air pollution, filling wetlands, etc.—and "undesirable and sick" people. These tended to be piecemeal interventions, with the exception of the sanitary survey, and rarely addressed consumption patterns that led to environmental wastes. For sanitarians, the local solution to pollution was removal and dilution, but the downstream environmental health impacts were ignored. While specific housing reforms, such as bathrooms, ventilation, and fire escapes improved health, they were rarely accompanied by demands for the construction of new public housing for the poor (Marcuse 1980). Most reforms were grounded in the belief that advancements in science and technology could provide physical improvements that would make "pathogenic" urban environments and the "immoral" slum-dwellers more orderly and healthy (Fairfield 1994). Professional white elites, from sanitary engineers to settlement house workers, rarely sought to organize a grassroots multiracial "urban environmental health" social movement or merge their work with concurrent movements for occupational health and safety and environmental conservation (Gottlieb 1993; Merchant 1985; Rosner and Markowitz 1985).

1900–1920s: GERM THEORY AND THE RATIONAL CITY

By the turn of the new century, it was well known in public health that both miasma and contagion failed to explain certain aspects of urban health, such as why, with ubiquitous filth, epidemics only occurred sometimes and in some places. Contagion offered a theory of how disease traveled, but not where disease came from. By this time, the driving ideology in public health shifted to *germ theory,* which stated that microbes were the specific agents that caused infectious disease (Susser and Susser 1996). Treatment and disease management began to supercede strategies of physically removing harms and public health shifted toward specific interventions, such as immunizations and the chlorination of drinking water to kill disease-carrying microbes. While these new interventions were administered by the "new public health professionals"—namely, biologists, chemists, and physicians—some social reforms aimed at improving health continued. For example, organized labor achieved significant gains in the workplace after the devastating fire in 1911 at the Triangle Shirtwaist Company in New York City, ushering in worker compensation laws, rules on child labor, the eight-hour workday and other social safety-net guarantees (Rosner and Markowitz 1985).

Neighborhood Health Centers

During the early years of the twentieth century, power over urban programs shifted from the federal government and state capitals to municipal govern-

By the turn of the new century, it was well known in public health that both miasma and contagion failed to explain certain aspects of urban health, such as why, with ubiquitous filth, epidemics only occurred sometimes and in some places.

In his 1909 book, An Introduction to City Planning: Democracy's Challenge to the American City, *Benjamin Clarke Marsh argued that the planning profession ought to be judged on whether interventions improve the health of the least-well-off city dwellers, not on designing aesthetically pleasing and efficient cities.*

ments. One example of this "home-rule" shift was the creation of neighborhood health centers, which were financed by federal matching grants through the Maternity and Infancy Protection Act, also known as the Sheppard-Towner Act (Rosen 1971). These centers attempted to bring clinical and social services to the poor, instead of forcing needy residents to travel to far-away central offices. Health centers were started in predominantly immigrant neighborhoods of Milwaukee and Philadelphia, the Mohawk-Brighton district of Cincinnati, New York's Lower East Side, and the West End of Boston. One of the only community health centers to serve African-Americans was started in Atlanta by a women's club called The Neighborhood Union.

A central feature of the health center was the creation of block committees with community representatives. These committees met regularly and provided an opportunity for residents to directly participate in community affairs, while also using the professional skills of the health center's physicians and nurses (Sparer 1971). Block workers represented residents and visited families, keeping them in touch with center programs and raising their concerns at meetings (Kreidler 1919). Another committee run by the health center, the occupational council, organized local business and professional groups and gathered their input and support for the work of the center. Both committees acted as neighborhood planning bodies since no new activities were undertaken in the neighborhood until they had the support of the two councils (Gillette 1983).

While merging social and physical planning with health services for the poor, neighborhood health centers declined rapidly after World War I. Criticism by physicians and the powerful American Medical Association, which accused the centers of practicing "socialized medicine," diminished their political and financial support (Rosen 1971). Federal matching funding for neighborhood health centers ended when the Sheppard-Towner Act was allowed to expire in 1929.

The Emergence of Professional Planning

The private sector saw an opportunity to profit after the 1893 World's Columbian Exposition in Chicago and took the lead in promoting a citywide plan to construct a network of parks, major roads, public buildings, art, and an amusement park (Hall 1996). The plan, released in 1909 by Daniel Burnham and Edward Bennett, became known as the *Plan of Chicago* and ushered in the City Beautiful movement that defined early American planning (Peterson 2003). A new professional class of city planners emerged, embraced the idea of comprehensive planning, and rejected the piecemeal approach of earlier reformers in favor of a belief that rational physical designs would eventually bring social and moral improvement to blighted urban areas (Peterson 2003).

Planning the beautiful and efficient city would soon become the responsibility of technically trained professionals, but debate surfaced over whether the field should concern itself with public health. Benjamin Marsh, the leader of the Committee on the Congestion of Population (CCP), argued that the new profession ought to concern itself with what he thought caused urban problems, including private property rights, inadequate public housing, and an inattention to the health of the poor (Marsh 1909). In his 1909 book, *An Introduction to City Planning: Democracy's Challenge to the American City*, Benjamin Clarke Marsh stated that the planning profession ought to be judged on whether interventions improve the health of the least-well-off city dwellers, not on designing aesthetically pleasing and efficient cities, noting:

> [N]o city is more healthy than the highest death rate in any ward or block and...no city is more beautiful than its most unsightly tenement. The back yard of a city and not its front lawn is the real criterion for its standards and its efficiency.... It compels a departure from the doctrine that government should not assume any functions aside from its primitive and restrictive

activities and boldly demands the interest and effort of the government to preserve the health, morals and efficiency of the citizens equal to the effort and the zeal which is now expended in the futile task of trying to make amends for the exploitation by private citizens and the wanton disregard of the rights of many. (Marsh 1909, 27)

However, the views of Marsh and the CCP were challenged by Frederick Law Olmsted Jr., then president of the National Conference on City Planning, who would later state in his keynote address at the second national conference that the profession was a "forum" for all those involved with the physical shaping of cities, not just for addressing the needs of the poor (Olmsted Jr. 1910). The views of the CCP were increasingly marginalized. By the third professional conference in 1911, the "problems of congestion" part of the title had been dropped, and by the fifth national conference in 1913, entitled "The City Scientific," Olmsted Jr. and his supporters had successfully defined the burgeoning field as technocratic, and professionals were debating how to incorporate new scientific and technical tools into their practice of analyzing and designing efficient cities (Fairfield 1994; Petersen 2003).

"Zoning was the heaven-sent nostrum for sick cities, the wonder drug of the planners, the balm sought by lending institutions and householders alike."

Zoning and Public Health

Under pressure from private land owners to prevent noxious industries from locating in residential districts or near exclusive shopping areas where they had invested, American city planners extended Taylorist notions of scientific efficiency in adopting a hierarchical ordering of land uses (Ford 1915). American zoning ordinances borrowed from the German ideas that divided cities by districts based on land use and housing type and built on nuisance laws used to protect public health by limiting odors, smoke, fumes, noises, and other noxious emissions from urban industries (Logan 1976). New York City developed the first citywide zoning code in 1916 that specified building heights and setbacks and created residential, commercial, and industrial zones.

Zoning ordinances were couched as both protecting public health and benefiting private land owners. As Scott (1971, 192) notes, "zoning was the heaven-sent nostrum for sick cities, the wonder drug of the planners, the balm sought by lending institutions and householders alike." In practice, zoning tended to preserve the status quo through "exclusionary" zoning and deed restrictions, or restrictive covenants, both acting to perpetuate Jim Crow segregation (Babcock 1966, 116). Zoning was also used by suburban planners to mandate minimum lot size, housing type, and house size in order to keep out low-income people, the majority of whom were immigrants and southern African-Americans coming north during the Great Migration (Haar and Kayden 1989). Extending Scott's (1971) use of health metaphors, zoning effectively "immunized" wealthy and white populations from having the poor and African-Americans live in their neighborhoods.

The Neighborhood Unit

Another land-use idea from this era, also couched as a way to improve the quality of urban life and bring more order to American cities, was the "neighborhood unit" concept. The neighborhood unit, proposed by Clarence Perry, was a design scheme of single-family lots, anchored around a primary school, designed for no more than 5,000 people (Perry 1929, 98). Reflecting an urban form similar to the Garden City ideal, the interior of the neighborhood unit consisted of a street pattern that encouraged pedestrian circulation and reduced street congestion caused by automobiles, while the periphery of the unit consisted of businesses located at traffic intersections. While Perry's scheme was hailed as a design that might optimize space for the efficient delivery of services, provide for a safe residential environment, and encourage the social values of the day, the neighborhood unit was also criticized by some as a physical design that ignored the social, economic, and political complexities of urban living and a plan that would ultimately promote economic residential segregation (Isaacs 1948). For more on Perry, including a drawing of his neighborhood unit, see Chapter 5 in this PAS Report.

1930s–1950s: THE BIOMEDICAL MODEL AND PATHOGENIC CITY

The federal insurance of home mortgages systematically ignored the plight of existing urban residents by refusing to insure mortgages for older houses, effectively "redlining" inner-city neighborhoods out of the program.

The driving theory in public health would shift again during the pre-WWII era to the *biomedical model* of disease. This model attributes morbidity and mortality to molecular-level pathogens brought about by individual life-styles, behaviors, hereditary biology, or genetics, and it altered attention in the field to personal "risk factors," such as smoking, diet, and exercise (Susser and Susser 1996). However, New Deal programs kept public health linked to engineering and planning by creating federal agencies to rebuild public health infrastructure, such as drinking water and sewer systems, hospitals, and new sources of electricity (Grey 1999). The New Deal also provided federal funding for municipal planning and health departments, ushering in the era of the "bureaucratic city" in which a new set of impersonal public institutions, staffed by newly credentialed professionals, laid claim to expert interventions. As separate municipal departments for everything from sanitation to sewerage to smoke control were created, distinct professionals and academic "silos" followed (Peterson 2003).

Public Health and the Neighborhood Unit

Perry's neighborhood unit idea took hold with planners, developers, and, in perhaps the most striking linkage between planning and public health of the early twentieth century, the American Public Health Association's (APHA) Committee on the Hygiene of Housing. The APHA committee adopted the neighborhood unit design scheme as the basis for two reports; one, in 1938, *Basic Principles of Healthful Housing*, and a second in 1948, *Planning the Neighborhood*. The latter document set standards for the "environment of residential areas," defined as "the area served by an elementary school," and emphasized that:

> No perfection in the building or equipment of the home can compensate for an environment which lacks the amenities essential for decent living. We must build not merely homes but neighborhoods if we are to build wisely for the future of America…[T]he effects of substandard environment extends beyond direct threats to physiological health, and involves…significant detriments to mental and emotional well-being. (APHA 1948, vi-vii)

Significantly, both the 1938 and 1948 documents recognized the existence and persistence of health disparities in poor neighborhoods and the how stigma might influence health status:

> [T]he mere elimination of specific hazards in poor neighborhoods falls short of the real goal of planning an environment which will foster a healthy and normal family life…a sense of inferiority due to living in a substandard home may often be a more serious health menace then any unsanitary condition associated with housing. (APHA 1948, vii)

Yet, the APHA committee stopped short of recognizing that widespread residential segregation might contribute to poor health, stating: "Further research is needed to determine to what extent housing segregation or housing aggregation of differing population groups may create mental tensions or otherwise affect health" (APHA 1948, 2).

Banerjee and Baer (1984, 24–5), in a detailed review of *Planning the Neighborhood*, observed that the APHA guidelines were instantly influential because most practitioners presumed that the design standards it offered linked the built environment with health when no other similar standards existed, even though there was no measurement technology at the time to confirm the "numerical precision" contained in the report. Other critics of *Planning the Neighborhood* challenged its physical deterministic orientation. Yet, as Fischler (1998, 390) has noted, the APHA adoption of the neighborhood unit and publication of specific healthy design standards "represent the culmination of a search for scientific methods to secure collective well-being."

Housing and Urban Renewal

Another set of policies geared toward housing, slum removal, and highway construction would have an even greater impact on the health of urban populations during this era (Hirsh 1983; Mohl 2000). By 1931, a group of influential women, led by Catherine Bauer, Mary Simkhovitch, and Edith Elmer Wood, organized the National Public Housing Conference (Peterson 2003). Drawing inspiration from European public housing programs, these women argued for a greater federal government role in building housing for the poor that was safe, affordable, and constructed in modernist, high-rise buildings on super-blocks, and in order to build this housing, existing slums had to be cleared.

The federal insurance of home mortgages began in 1934 through the Federal Housing Administration (FHA), and also systematically ignored the plight of existing urban residents by refusing to insure mortgages for older houses, effectively "redlining" inner-city neighborhoods out of the program (Fishman 2000). White racism in housing was perpetuated by the planning field's acceptance and perpetuation of this de facto policy of segregation (Hirsh 1983). The Housing Act of 1949 would later establish the idea of urban renewal where municipalities began razing "slum" neighborhoods and displacing thousands of poor, largely African-American residents.

Urban renewal was a program and theory that aimed to remove downtown blight—still viewed as the cause of moral evil and the breeding ground for disease—and rebuild whole sections of the city using the best of modern technology and scientifically rational design (Fishman 2000). Yet, urban renewal tended to only increase poverty for residents of poor neighborhoods because their homes were replaced with either inadequate public housing or, as was more often the case, private real estate developers acquired the downtown land cheaply and opted not to build new housing but expensive, high-rise, office towers (Weiss 1980). Not only were neighborhoods physically fractured, but social and emotional ties, trust and notions of collective efficacy, particularly for African-Americans, were also severed by urban renewal (Fullilove 2004). Shut out from most new suburbs, African-Americans were denied other health benefits that can come with home ownership, such as capital accumulation, access to better-funded schools, and participation in the growing suburban economy. By the 1956 passage of the Federal Aid Highway Act, the field of planning had not only ignored the public health impacts of its programs, but had perpetuated the widespread destruction of the nation's poorest inner-city neighborhoods (Mohl 2000).

1960s–1980s: CRISIS AND THE ACTIVIST CITY

By the 1960s, planning was grappling with widespread social unrest, and the field was hard-pressed to respond to activists' claims that large-scale public development projects and modernist designs that accompanied urban renewal projects were not any better than piecemeal changes that built on the existing fabric of older neighborhoods (Goodman 1972). Activists also challenged public health professionals to address why, in the face of rising economic prosperity and improvements in medical technology, inequalities in

Activists challenged public health professionals to address why, in the face of rising economic prosperity and improvements in medical technology, inequalities in health persisted particularly for the urban poor and people of color,

health persisted particularly for the urban poor and people of color (Krieger 2000). For example, in 1960 the infant mortality rate was 44.3 per 1,000 for African-American babies and 29.2 for whites (Satcher et al. 2005, 459).

Civil Rights activists organized in urban areas to link social, environmental, and health justice. For example, the Young Lords, a group of New York City Puerto Rican activists in "El Barrio" or East Harlem, organized street cleanups after the sanitation department refused to collect neighborhood garbage for weeks. The group convinced local health professionals to train lay residents in the techniques of door-to-door lead-poisoning screening and tuberculosis testing (Abramson et al. 1971). The Lords started day care programs in local churches, provided breakfast in neighborhood schools, organized tenants to demand housing improvements, and occupied a neighborhood hospital to highlight its inadequate service to the local population (Melendez 2003).

The key challenge for reconnecting planning and public health in the twenty-first century is to learn from each field's history and jointly develop strategies that address the root causes of poor health, not just devise interventions aimed at specific diseases or individual behaviors.

By 1970, the Nixon Administration began redirecting resources away from inner cities to the suburbs through block grants, dismantling Model Cities programs, and instituting "benign neglect," a policy of not responding to emergency alarms in poor minority neighborhoods. ("Benign neglect" was proposed by Daniel Patrick Moynihan, Nixon's advisor on urban and social policy, in his 1970 memo reprinted in the *New York Times* on January 30, 1970, *Text of the Moynihan memorandum on the status of negroes*.)

New York City adopted a *de facto* policy of "planned shrinkage," where essential services, such as libraries, fire protection, and public transportation were withdrawn from designated "sick" neighborhoods and redirected to "healthier" ones (Fried 1976; Roberts 1991). As ghettos were left to burn, the twentieth century's most significant environmental health legislation was passed, including the creation of the Environmental Protection Agency, the Occupational Health and Safety Administration, and the National Environmental Policy, Clean Air, and Clean Water Acts. A proposed National Land Use Planning Act was defeated in 1974, but its debate as "jobs versus the environment" acted to split a coalition of urban African-American activists that would hold through much of the next two decades (Weir 2000). However, by the end of this era, the Centers for Disease Control recognized that improving urban health required attention to more than just the physical characteristics of neighborhoods; it also demanded attention to the social and psychological implications of housing, removal, and relocation (Hinkle and Loring 1977).

1990s–TWENTY-FIRST CENTURY: EMERGING PARADIGMS

The 1988 release of the Institute of Medicine's Committee for the Study of the Future of Public Health report made it clear that leaders in the field agreed the nation's public health activities were in disarray and the field needed to refocus its efforts to address the growing inequalities in health across population groups (IOM 1988). By the 1990s, public health research in the UK, Canada, and the U.S. began to reconceptualize explanations for the *distribution* of disease across populations in order to explain health disparities, energizing the field of social epidemiology (Berkman and Kawachi 2000).

Social epidemiology, by emphasizing *distribution* as distinct from *causation*, pushed public health to reconsider how poverty, economic inequality, stress, discrimination, and social capital become "biologically embodied" and helped explain persistent patterns of inequitable distributions of disease and well-being across different population groups and geographic areas (Krieger 2000). By the end of the twentieth century, a split emerged in public health between those emphasizing the biomedical model and focusing on treating individual disease "risk factors," and the social epidemiologists who emphasized nineteenth century ideas of improving neighborhood conditions, eliminating poverty, and enhancing social resources for health (Fitzpatrick and LaGory 2000; Geronimus 2000; Klinenberg 2002).

Reconnecting the Fields for the Twenty-first Century

The key challenge for reconnecting planning and public health in the twenty-first century is to learn from each field's history and jointly develop strategies that address the *root causes* of poor health, not just devise interventions aimed at specific diseases or individual behaviors. As this brief history has shown, effective reconnection efforts must be attentive to the political questions of governance, existing issue framings, and the reliance on professional scientific knowledge for social problem solving. Grappling with the political challenges of reconnecting the fields demands that, for instance, planners experiment with new institutional designs that can handle cross-disciplinary conflicts over political power, social justice, and health values, such as when a state or private-sector-sponsored development project clashes with the health objectives of a local community. Planners will also need to critically question the adequacy of existing norms and institutions that help determine how practitioners use or abuse power, respond to or even resist market forces, work to empower some groups and disempower others, promote multiparty decision making, or simply rationalize decisions already made.

Reconnecting through Precaution and Prevention

The first lesson from the histories of planning and public health is that removal and displacement of "problems" does not necessarily improve urban health and may leave the most vulnerable groups and places worse off. For example, Fullilove (2004) suggests that residential upheaval and lack of resettlement from urban renewal programs continue to have mental and physical health impacts on African-Americans. Environmental justice researchers note that the historic removal and displacement of environmental toxics tended to concentrate hazardous burdens in low income and minority communities (Bullard 1994; Hurley 1995). Instead of removal and displacement, the precautionary principle, now widely used to guide environmental health decision making in Europe (Commission of European Communities 2000), may be a more appropriate social justice frame through which to grapple with twenty-first century challenges for reconnecting urban planning and public health. A forthcoming PAS Report in summer 2007 will address the history and current practice of environmental justice in greater detail.

The precautionary principle is an analytic and decision-making framework that seeks to reduce or eliminate pathogenic exposures, to ecosystems and humans, by asking whether a toxin or proposed policy is needed, setting environmental and public health performance goals with impacted stakeholders, and collaboratively reviewing prevention scenarios, even in the absence of definitive proof of harm (Tickner and Geiser 2004). Drawing from the clinical notion of "first, do no harm," the precautionary principle challenges the current "command and control" environmental health regulatory model where the state is responsible for generating scientific proof of harm before taking regulatory action. Instead, the precautionary approach demands that preventive and protective action should be taken even in the face of uncertain science and that the burden of proof of safety rests with those who create risks. By requiring action in the face of uncertainty, the precautionary principle also demands that affected stakeholders explore actionable alternatives, often redirecting environmental health science and policy from describing problems to identifying solutions. The European Union has, in fact, institutionalized the precautionary and alternatives assessment processes suggested here (Cone 2005).

The precautionary approach demands that preventive and protective action should be taken even in the face of uncertain science and that the burden of proof of safety rests with those who create risks.

An overreliance on technological solutions and physical designs, without accompanying institutional change, fails to protect the most vulnerable population groups.

Health impact assessment (HIA) is one example of a precautionary practice that might link planning and public health. Now widely used for healthy urban planning in Europe, HIA is both an analytic tool and political process that might bring together the built and social environmental factors that influence urban health (Barnes and Scott-Samuel 2002). For example, the San Francisco Department of Public Health (SFDPH) has used HIA to assess a proposed living wage ordinance, new housing proposals, and rezoning plans. The agency has also used HIA to promote social justice by evaluating how these projects might distribute health impacts (both positive and negative) across the population, if potential impacts will be shared unequally across the population, if the potential differential health impacts are avoidable and unfair—that is, inequitable, and if inequities are likely, what alternative scenarios are possible (Bhatia 2003). While no panacea, experiments with HIA in San Francisco and Europe suggest it offers a process for bringing together city agencies that traditionally had not worked together, such as public health, economic development, planning, and youth services, suggesting it may be one way to break down "disciplinary silos" and other institutional barriers confronting efforts to reconnect planning and public health.

Reconnecting planning and public health in the twenty-first century will also have to find new ways to prevent adverse health impacts of housing policies. The Progressive Era strategy of physically improving urban housing is a necessary but insufficient strategy because it ignores the social and regional health impacts of housing policies. For instance, as affordable housing decreases, low-income populations are not only forced to accept substandard and hazardous living conditions, which can trigger asthma and increase lead-poisoning, but they may also be forced to relocate to areas far away from social and family support networks or become homeless (Krieger and Higgins 2002). One particular housing program, the Moving to Opportunity Program (MTO), sponsored by the U.S. Department of Housing and Urban Development, is an example of a strategy that runs the risk of repeating the missteps of historic removal programs. While early reports suggest that some members of the African-American inner-city families that were relocated to white suburbs have experienced acute health improvements, such as fewer asthma attacks, temporary reductions in obesity, and decreased anxiety for female youths, the longer-term benefits are less clear (Kling et al. 2004). For instance, Kling et al. (2004) report that after a year in their new surroundings, male youth in the MTO program were more likely to engage in risky behavior, experience more physical and mental health problems, and adults experience no net gains in general health or reductions in hypertension. Like earlier urban removal schemes, the MTO program runs the risk of skirting the political issue of racism that led to urban ghettos, offers no benefits to ghetto residents left behind, limits discourse over desegregation programs, and fails to acknowledge the social and cultural strengths of urban African-American neighborhoods that can be protective and healthy, such as kin care networks.

Finally, a prevention and precaution framework might offer an alternative to another inner-city people removal strategy: incarceration (Wacquant 2002). American jail populations are disproportionately made up of young, urban, African-American and Latino men—the same groups that have the poorest health in the U.S. Incarceration has created a planning and public health challenge by spatially concentrating both the removal of young men from families and the workforce, and the social stress that accompanies inmates' return to their neighborhoods. For instance, in New York City, almost 70 percent of the 2002 jail population came from one of three neighborhoods—the South Bronx, Harlem, and Central Brooklyn—more than half are released and return to jail within the same year, and the city spends more than $92,000 per year to incarcerate one person (Bloomberg 2003; NYC DOC 2003). The constant cycle of incarceration and reentry in New York and other urban areas has brought the health issues of prisons into the neighborhood, including infectious disease, addiction, mental health problems, and routine physical violence. Yet, returning inmates face homelessness, family evictions from public housing, denial of food stamps, terminated Medicaid benefits, and regular workplace discrimination (Black and Cho 2004). In the twenty-first century, incarceration and reentry must become planning and public health issues so that, for instance, municipal funds are redirected to provide the place-based housing, education, employment, and social services necessary to prevent recidivism and reduce the spatial impacts of incarceration.

New Institution Building

A second set of related lessons from the histories of planning and public health is that an overreliance on technological solutions and physical designs, without accompanying institutional change, fails to protect the most vulnerable population groups. Planners might aim to develop "urban health and sustainability" programs that learn from successful adaptive management schemes now used to manage natural resources, such as Habitat Conservation Plans (HCP). Under these programs, instead of one-size-fits-all rules, interventions are adjusted over time as new technologies emerge, learning occurs, and continuous monitoring reveals how actual conditions are changing. Another lesson is that economic development in the absence of community-based institutions may fail to improve living conditions. Community-based institutions can help ensure that the benefits of economic development are distributed to meet the needs of local people. For example, a coalition of community-based organizations called the Figueroa Corridor Coalition successfully negotiated a community benefit agreement (CBA) with the Los Angeles Arena Land Company, a private developer, over the Staples Center Phase II project in downtown Los Angeles (Goodno 2004). The CBA is a legally binding agreement guaranteeing that the developer include affordable housing and public amenities, such as new parks, and that the new commercial establishments hire local residents at a living wage (Gross et al. 2002). Reminiscent of struggles for early twentieth century workplace and neighborhood improvements, organized labor unions are acting as integral partners in shaping these agreements, recognizing that their members increasingly come from low-income communities and are working in service-sector jobs.

Tempering Professional Models with Lay Expertise

A final lesson from the histories of planning and public health is that when interventions ignore what local people know, how they move through the world, and their subjective experiences with illness and their environment, the interventions ultimately fail (Scott 1998). Local knowledge, including the experiences and narratives shared by populations living with persistent hazardous exposures, chronic diseases, and social marginalization, is a valuable form of "expertise" that can improve scientific analyses, the relevance of health-promoting interventions, and the democratic character of public decisions (Corburn 2003). Drawing from the lessons of the neighborhood health center movement, twenty-first century planning and public health might reembrace local knowledge by promoting and supporting networks of community health workers (CHWs).

Often called *promotoras de salud*, CHWs are frontline lay health outreach workers that organize neighborhood residents around health issues and provide health education, basic disease screening, and translation services. CHWs often act as the bridge builders between poor, minority, and immigrant

When interventions ignore what local people know, how they move through the world, and their subjective experiences with illness and their environment, the interventions ultimately fail.

communities and professional health services and institutions. Since CHWs live in the places within which they work, they have a keen awareness of local culture and practices and often have experience of how macrosocial structures impact the daily lives of local residents. Ultimately, CHWs tap local knowledge to improve health by building community; stimulating informal networks, formal associations, and other connections between socially dissimilar persons or groups that can be crucial for securing both immediate health promoting resources and organizing long-term policy advocacy coalitions (Satterfield et al. 2002).

REINTEGRATING PLANNING AND PUBLIC HEALTH FOR THE TWENTY-FIRST CENTURY

This chapter has aimed to both critically review the histories of American urban planning and public health, and, by drawing lessons from this review, suggest strategies to reconnect the fields to confront twenty-first century challenges. The contemporary challenges for reconnecting the fields are daunting—global spread of disease, transboundary environmental pollution, burgeoning urban and slum populations, and increasing health disparities mirroring widening class inequalities. As momentum for the reconnection effort builds, as reflected in recent journal issues, conferences, government, and foundation efforts, the lessons from each fields' historic missteps ought to be given close scrutiny.

The recommendations offered here should also be viewed in a comparative perspective, since they reflect experiments aimed at "healthy urban planning" from around the world. For instance, the World Health Organization's City Action Group on Healthy Urban Planning (www.euro.who.int/document/e82657.pdf) and the UK Office of the Deputy Prime Minister's Creating Sustainable Communities initiative (www.odpm.gov.uk) are both principally focused on how to reverse social exclusion and inequality more generally through the design of new collaborative governance schemes, state regulations, and building nongovernmental capacity. In the UK, London and Merseyside are using HIA to address planning and development decisions (Scott-Samuel et al. 1998). Efforts to upgrade slums in developing countries, including strategies for achieving the Millennium Development Goals, explicitly call for the inclusion of local knowledge (Sachs 2003). Finally, the most successful campaign to reduce AIDS in Haiti, the poorest country with the highest rate of HIV infection, was designed around networks of CHWs (Farmer 1999).

Contemporary efforts to reconnect planning and public health can learn from the past to understand how current trends gained resonance and what alternative futures are possible. Alternative paradigms can be both practical and socially just, as the examples here suggest. However, since many of the recommendations are offered as frameworks, not specific guidance, more work needs to be done to evaluate which practices might work best in specific cultural and political contexts. Yet, as efforts to reconnect urban planning and public health move forward, a historic perspective is necessary to critically reengage with our roots and forge a twenty-first century urban health agenda.

CHAPTER 3 LIST OF REFERENCES

[*This List of References is supplemented by a Master Resource List at the end of this PAS Report.*]

Abramson, Michael et al. 1971. *Palante: Young Lords Party*. New York: McGraw-Hill.

APHA (American Public Health Association). 1948. *Planning the Neighborhood: Standards for Healthful Housing*. Chicago: Public Administration Service, Committee on the Hygiene of Housing.

Babcock, R. F. 1966. *The Zoning Game: Municipal Practices and Policies*. Madison: University of Wisconsin Press.

Barnes, R., and A. Scott-Samuel. 2002. "Health Impact Assessment and Inequalities." *Pan American Journal of Public Health* 11 (5/6): 449–53.

Berkman, L., and I. Kawachi. eds. 2000. *Social Epidemiology*. New York: Oxford University Press.

Bhatia, R. 2003. "Swimming Upstream in a Swift Current: Public Health Institutions and Inequality." In *Health and Social Justice*, edited by Richard Hofrichter. San Francisco: Jossey-Bass, 557–78.

Black, K., and R. Cho. 2004. *New Beginnings: The Need for Supportive Housing for Previously Incarcerated People*. New York: Coalition for Supportive Housing and Common Ground.

Bloomberg, M. 2003. *Mayor's Management Report, Fiscal Year 2003*. New York: Office of the Mayor.

Boyer, C. 1983. *Dreaming the Rational City: The Myth of American City Planning*. Cambridge: MIT Press.

Burrows, E.G., and M. Wallace. 1999. *Gotham: A History of New York City to 1898*. New York: Oxford University Press.

CDC (Centers for Disease Control and Prevention). 2004. *Designing and Building Healthy Places*. http://www.cdc.gov/healthyplaces/

Cone, M. 2005. "Europe's Rules Forcing U.S. Firms to Clean Up." *Los Angeles Times*, 16 May, Part A:1.

Corburn, J. 2005. *Street Science: Community Knowledge and Environmental Health Justice*. Cambridge: The MIT Press.

Dannenberg, A. L., Bhatia, R. Cole, B.L. et al. 2006. "Growing the Field of Health Impact Assessment in the United States: An Agenda for Research and Practice." *American Journal of Public Health* 96: 262–70.

Duffy, J. 1990. *The Sanitarians: A History of American Public Health*. Chicago: University of Illinois Press.

Duhl, L. J., and A. K. Sanchez. 1999. *Healthy Cities and the City Planning Process*. http://www.who.dk/document/e67843.pdf.

Fairfield, J. D. 1994. "The Scientific Management of Urban Space: Professional City Planning and the Legacy of Progressive Reform." *Journal of Urban History* 20: 179–204.

Farmer, P. 1999. *Infections and Inequalities: The Modern Plagues*. Berkeley: University of California Press.

Fischler, R. 1998. "For a Genealogy of Planning." *Planning Perspectives* 13, no. 4: 389–410.

Fishman, R. ed. 2000. *The American Planning Tradition: Culture and Policy*. Washington, D.C.: Woodrow Wilson Center Press.

Fitzpatrick, K., and M. LaGory. 2000. *Unhealthy Places: The Ecology of Risk in The Urban Landscape*. London: Routledge

Ford, G. B. 1915. *The City Scientific. Proceedings of the Fifth National Conference in City Planning*, 31-39.

Fox, D. M., R.J. Jackson, and J.A. Barondess. 2003. "Health and the Built Environment." *Journal of Urban Health* 80, no. 4: 534–35.

Fried, J. 1976. "City's Housing Administrator Proposes "Planned Shrinkage" of Some Slums. *New York Times*, 3 February, B1.

Frumkin, H. 2002. "Urban Sprawl and Public Health." *Public Health Reports* 117, 201–17.

Fullilove, M. T. 2004. *Root Shock: How Tearing Up City Neighborhoods Hurts America and What We Can Do about It*. New York: Ballantine.

Geronimus, A T. 2000. "To Mitigate, Resist, or Undo: Addressing Structural Influences on the Health of Urban Populations." *American Journal of Public Health* 90, 867–72.

Gillette Jr., H. 1983. "The Evolution of Neighborhood Planning: From the Progressive Era to the 1949 Housing Act." *Journal of Urban History* 9, no. 4: 421–44.

Goodman, R. 1971. *After the Planners*. New York: Simon & Schuster.

Goodno, J. B. 2004. "Feet to the Fire." *Planning* 70, no. 4: 14–19.

Gottlieb, R. 1993. *Forcing the Spring: The Transformation of the American Environmental Movement*. Washington D.C.: Island Press.

Gross, J., G. LeRoy, and M. Janis-Aparicio. 2002. *Community Benefit Agreements: Making Development Projects Accountable*. Washington, D.C.: Good Jobs First and the California Public Subsidies Project. http://www.goodjobsfirst.org/pdf/cba2005final.pdf

Haar, C. M., and J.S. Kayden. eds. 1989. *Zoning and the American Dream: Promises Still to Keep*. Chicago: Planners Press.

Hall, P. 1996. *Cities of Tomorrow: An Intellectual History of Urban Planning and Design in the Twentieth Century*. Revised edition. Oxford: Blackwell.

Hinkle L.E., and W.C. Loring. eds. 1977. *The Effect of the Man-Made Environment on Health and Behavior*. Publication #CDC 77-8318. Atlanta, Ga.: Centers for Disease Control

Hirsh, A. R. 1983. *Making the Second Ghetto: Race and Housing in Chicago, 1940-1960*. Cambridge, Mass.: Cambridge University Press.

Hull-House, Residents of. 1895. *Hull House Maps and Papers*. New York: Thomas Y. Crowell & Co.

Hurley, A. 1995. *Environmental Inequalities: Class, Race, and Industrial Pollution in Gary, Indiana, 1945-1980*. Chapel Hill: University of North Carolina Press.

IOM (Institute of Medicine). 1988. *The Future of Public Health*. Washington, DC: National Academy Press.

Killingsworth, R., J. Earp, and R. Moore. 2003. "Supporting Health through Design: Challenges and Opportunities." *American Journal of Health Promotion* 18, no. 1: 1–2.

Klinenberg, E. 2002. *Heat Wave: A Social Autopsy of Disaster in Chicago*. University of Chicago Press

Kling, J.R., J.B. Liebman, L.F. Katz, & L. Sanbonmatsu. 2004. "Moving To Opportunity and Tranquility: Neighborhood Effects on Adult Economic Self –Sufficiency and Health from a Randomized Housing Voucher Experiment." Princeton University. www.wws.princeton.edu/kling/mto/481.pdf.

Krieger, J., and D.L. Higgins. 2002. "Housing and Health: Time and Again for Public Health Action." *American Journal of Public Health* 92, no. 5: 758–68.

Krieger, N. 2000. "Epidemiology and Social Sciences: Toward a Critical Reengagement in the 21st Century." Epidemiologic Reviews 22: 155–63.

Logan, T. 1976. "The Americanization of German Zoning." *Journal of the American Institute of Planning* 42, no. 4: 377–85.

Lubove, R. 1974. *The Progressives and the Slums: Tenement House Reform in New York City, 1870-1917*. Westport: Greenwood.

Marcuse, P. 1980. "Housing Policy and City Planning: The Puzzling Split in the United States, 1893-1931. In *Shaping an Urban World*, edited by G.E. Cherry. London: Mansell, 23–58.

Markel, H. 1997. *Quarantine! East European Jewish Immigrants and the New York City Epidemics of 1892*. Baltimore: Johns Hopkins University Press.

Marsh, B. 1909 [1974]. *An Introduction to City Planning: Democracy's Challenge to the American City*. New York: Ayer Company Publishing.

Melendez, M. 2003. *We Took the streets: Fighting for Latino Rights with the Young Lords*. New York: St. Martin's Press.

Melosi, M.V. 1973. "'Out of Sight, Out of Mind:' The Environment and Disposal of Municipal Refuse, 1860-1920." *Historian* 35: 629–40.

Melosi, M. 2000. *The Sanitary City: Urban Infrastructure in America from Colonial Times to the Present*. Baltimore: Johns Hopkins University Press.

Merchant, C. 1985. "The Women of the Progressive Conservation Crusade: 1900 – 1915." In *Environmental History: Critical Issues in Comparative Perspective*, edited by K.E. Bailes. New York: New York University Press, 153–75.

Mohl, R.A. 2000. "Planned Destruction: The Interstates and Central City Housing." In *From Tenements to the Taylor Homes*, edited by J. F. Bauman, R. Biles, and K.M. Szylvian. University Park: Pennsylvania State University Press, 226–45.

Mullan, F. 1989. *Plagues and Politics: The Story of the United States Public Health Service*. New York: Basic Books.

National Association of County and City Health Officials (NACCHO). 2004. *Integrating Public Health into Land Use Decision-Making*. http://www.naccho.org/project84.cfm.

New York City, Department of Correction (DOC). 2003. *Annual Report*. New York.

Olmsted Jr., F.L. 1910. "City Planning: An Introductory Address." *American Civic Association* 2, no. 4: 1–30.

Perry, C. A. 1929. "City Planning for Neighborhood Life." *Social Forces* 8, no. 1: 98–100.

Peterson, J. 2003. *The Birth of City Planning in the United States, 1840-1917*. Baltimore, Md.: Johns Hopkins University Press.

_____. 1979. "The Impact of Sanitary Reform upon American Urban Planning, 1840-1890." *Journal of Social History* 13: 83–103.

RWJF (Robert Wood Johnson Foundation). 2004. *Active Living by Design Program*. http://www.activelivingbydesign.org

Roberts, S. 1991. "A Critical Evaluation of the City Life Cycle Idea." *Urban Geography* 12: 431–49.

Rosen, G. 1971. "The First Neighborhood Health Center Movement—Its Rise and Fall." *American Journal of Public Health* 61: 1,620–37.

Rosen, G. 1993. *A History of Public Health*. Expanded edition. Baltimore, Md.: Johns Hopkins Press.

Rosner, D., and G. Markowitz. 1985. "The Early Movement for Occupational Safety and Health." In *Sickness and Health in America*, edited by J.W. Leavitt and R.L. Numbers. Madison:University of Wisconsin Press, 507–21.

Sachs, J. D. 2003. "The New Urban Planning." *Development Outreach* (November). http://www1.worldbank.org/devoutreach/nov03/article.asp?id=220

Satcher, D., G.E. Fryer, Jr., J. McCann, A. Troutman, S. H. Woolf, G. Rust. 2005. "What If We Were Equal? A Comparison of the Black-White Mortality Gap in 1960 and 2000." *Health Affairs* 24, no. 2: 459–64.

Satterfield, D. 2002. "The 'In-Between People': Participation of Community Health Representatives in Diabetes Prevention and Care in American Indian and Alaska Native communities." *Health Promotion Practice* 3, no. 2: 166–75.

Scott, J. 1998. *Seeing Like a State: How Certain Schemes To Improve the Human Condition Have Failed*. New Haven, Conn.: Yale University Press.

Scott, M. 1971. *American City Planning since 1890*. Berkeley: University of California.

Scott-Samuel A., M. Birley, and K. Ardern. 1998. *The Merseyside Guidelines for Health Impact Assessment.* Liverpool: Merseyside Health Impact Assessment Steering Group. http://www.liv.ac.uk/~mhb/publicat/merseygui/index.htm

Sparer, G., and J. Johnson. 1971. "Evaluation of OEO Neighborhood Health Centers." *American Journal of Public Health* 61, no. 5: 931–42.

Susser, M., and E. Susser. 1996. "Choosing a Future for Epidemiology: Eras and Paradigms. *American Journal of Public Health* 86, no. 5: 668–73.

Tarr, J.A. 1996. *The Search for the Ultimate Sink: Urban Pollution in Historical Perspective.* Akron, Ohio: University of Akron Press,

Tickner, J.A., and K. Geiser. 2004. "The Precautionary Principle Stimulus for Solutions and Alternatives-based Environmental Policy." *Environmental Impact Assessment Review* 24: 810–24.

Wacquant, L. 2002. "Deadly Symbiosis: Rethinking Race and Imprisonment in 21st Century America." *Boston Review.* http://www.bostonreview.net/BR27.2/wacquant.html

Weir, M. 2000. "Planning, Environmentalism and Urban Poverty." In *The American Planning Tradition: Culture and Policy*, edited byR. Fishman. Washington, D.C.: Woodrow Wilson Center Press, 193–215.

Weiss, M. A. 1980. "The Origins and Legacy of Urban Renewal. In *Urban and Regional Planning in an Age of Austerity*, edited byP. Clavel, J. Forester, and W. W. Goldsmith. New York: Pergamon Press, 53–80.

CHAPTER 4

Five Strategic Points of Intervention and Collaboration Between Planning and Public Health

By Marya Morris, AICP

and-use policies and land development in general directly affect numerous aspects of public and environmental health. APA has chosen to address these areas of common interest between planning and public health by looking at the points in the planning process where public health officials should have a stronger voice. In general, by involving local public health officials at the earliest stages of policy formation and keeping them involved in the planning process until changes are observable on the ground, we can create better plans that provide communities strong tools to protect and even improve health.

The framework that APA is using to promote an interdisciplinary, multi-objective approach to policy making and implementation is what we call the Five Strategic Points of Intervention:

1. Visioning and Goal Setting

2. Plans and Planning

3. Implementation Tools

4. Site Design and Development

5. Public Facility Siting and Capital Spending

Where the points of intervention are aimed at specific outcomes (e.g., revised plans that address the health impacts of land-use policies), we also recommend readers consider the tactical and process-oriented aspects of these interventions. To that end, we recognize these as the five strategic points of *collaboration* to drive the actual interventions.

THE FIRST POINT OF INTERVENTION: VISIONING AND GOAL SETTING

When a plan is being prepared or revised, planners call on a broad mix of stakeholders—the public, developers, builders, housing experts and advocates, transportation specialists, environmentalists, advocates for specific populations (e.g., the elderly or persons with a disability)—to provide input for the plan's goals, objectives, and strategies. Despite the breadth of this stakeholder list, public health professionals and advocates are not usually included. For communities to be successful in planning for and designing health-promoting, active, and accessible environments, planners will have to seek out public health professionals and include them at the very outset of planning processes.

At the initial visioning sessions, a planner or other representative of the coordinating agency gives an overview of the scope of issues. This is followed by a facilitated discussion, breakout groups, or some other type of session in which the public can say what it would like to see the plan contain, what it would not want it to contain, what changes to the built environment it would like to see happen, and what changes it does not want to occur. What emerges from these sessions is some consensus on shared values and a set of principles that provides a broad context within which planners establish the plan's goals.

Protecting and enhancing quality of life is a value that invariably arises in such visioning sessions. From the health profession's standpoint, it is a concept that relates directly to the health and physical well-being of individuals. But the quality-of-life discussion affecting land-use planning rarely addresses how the built environment—and the changes being proposed in whichever plan is being prepared—will either enhance or hinder the public's health. Instead, planners define quality of life by a broader set of factors (e.g., the impact of proposed changes on traffic congestion, housing affordability, loss of open space, children's safety outside their homes, availability of local services, and building or code enforcement).

The absence of health and physical activity representatives at visioning and plan preparation stages results in several missed opportunities. First, planners and public health practitioners could use such sessions to educate the public about how communities develop and the effect development patterns have on their mobility choices (e.g., whether they can walk, take transit, or must drive to where they are going) and their ability to be physically active when following their daily routines.

Second, the public health field has become a strong advocate for smart growth planning, bringing its expertise and support to built environment

For communities to be successful in planning for and designing health-promoting, active, and accessible environments, planners will have to seek out public health professionals and include them at the very outset of planning processes.

issues (e.g., compact, walkable neighborhoods, mixed use, street connectivity, traffic calming, parks, recreation and trails planning, reducing impervious surfaces, and supporting transit). The endorsement of these professionals can add significant political weight to the inclusion of health goals in a plan.

Beyond this opportunity for specific points of intervention in the planning process, planners and public health people should be collaborating routinely on areas of overlap—there is no reason to wait until a plan gets underway. In fact, to the extent that the two disciplines begin collaborating and sharing information formally or informally as a matter or course, the easier it will be to bring public health practitioners to the table when a planning process gets underway. To that end, the activities recommended here should not only be undertaken at the beginning of a planning process, but as a matter of routine.

Prior to the visioning sessions or workshops:

- Public health practitioners should convene to discuss obesity, physical inactivity, and other public health issues related to land use and the built environment.

- Public health professionals should make presentations to planning staff, planning commissioners, and other local officials to explain the connections between planning, community design, and health problems (e.g., obesity, physical activity, asthma, and waterborne disease and outbreaks).

- Public health practitioners can also educate land-use and transportation planners about the issues they as health professionals plan to bring to the table (e.g. pedestrian safety).

- Planners should brief local public health practitioners about what to expect in the planning process.

- Planners and public health officials can form a standing committee (i.e., a working group) that meets regularly on the relationship between health and the built environment. For example, this group could: a) keep up to date on issues of shared concern; b) pursue collaborative projects (e.g., conducting a community environmental health assessment); c) prepare for future planning processes; and d) monitor plan implementation to ensure that health and physical activity objectives are being met. (See also Chapter 6, Health Impact Assessment, for another example of a collaborative task.)

During the visioning process:

- Planners should extend invitations and encourage public health representatives to attend the public visioning and goal-setting sessions.

- Public health representatives should offer to chair or participate in advisory committees or work groups.

- Public health and planners should champion the inclusion of goals and objectives that explicitly relate to increasing opportunities for physical activity and reducing obesity.

- Planners should revisit smart growth goals and policies currently in place that support healthy communities.

THE SECOND POINT OF INTERVENTION: PLANS AND PLANNING

The specific goals for public health established in the visioning sessions or the early stages of a planning process can be conveyed in a plan in a number

Planners and public health people should be collaborating routinely on areas of overlap—there is no reason to wait until a plan gets underway.

of ways. How that is done will depend on the plan's overall format and the plan's focus (e.g., parks and open space, housing, transportation, etc.). The most effective way of ensuring that public health improvement is addressed by the plan is to make it one of the plan's overarching goals.

In addition to concisely worded goals, the plan can also include a narrative description of the relationship of planning to health. This would provide the public and other plan users with an explanation of the focus on health and physical activity, which will signify a new policy direction for most jurisdictions. In 2005, communities prepared hundreds of excellent plans that contain all that is necessary to achieve the smart growth goals of walkable streets and districts, the inclusion of bike lanes and trails, street connectivity, human-scale architecture, traffic calming, and many other measures but which never expressly address health as one of the plan goals. That is changing gradually. King County, Washington, and Orange County, Florida, in 2005 both incorporated explicit language in their plans making it clear that these plan policies are intended to be in furtherance of both smart growth and public health.

With the overarching goals in place, more targeted health-related objectives and policies can be incorporated into relevant plan elements (i.e., subsets of the plan that address specific issues; for example, land use, needed public health infrastructure, transportation, economic development, etc.) as well as the implementation program, or schedule, for the plan. For example, a broad goal to increase opportunities for people to be physically active as part of their daily routine could be carried forward by policies in the transportation element (among others) to require developers to install sidewalks on both sides of the street. A description of the importance of making it possible for people to make daily trips from home to work, school, or shopping would be well placed in a transportation element, a bicycle and pedestrian plan element, a trails element, and others.

Plan Content and Planning Process Interventions: How to Incorporate Health Objectives into Plans

The Comprehensive Plan

- Provide a narrative description of the rationale for addressing health and physical activity for all people in the comprehensive plan, including a description of how smart growth principles already being implemented in the community are supportive of active living.

- Develop overarching goals that tie cardiovascular health, safety, physical activity, and obesity to planning, community design, and land use.

- Establish more specific goals relating to health in each plan element or functional plan adopted as part of the comprehensive plan.

- Create an implementation schedule or program to achieve health-related goals that identifies which agency or organization will lead the implementation, prescribe the timeline, and pinpoint funding sources.

Special Area Plans, Neighborhood Plans, Redevelopment District Plans, Subarea Plans, and Functional Plans (Comprehensive Plan Elements or Chapters)

- Provide a narrative description of the planning/health issue as in the comprehensive plan but include specific language relevant to the physical planning area.

- Reference related goals in the comprehensive plan.

- Give a narrative description of the rationale for addressing health and physical activity in such a plan if it is a stand-alone plan (i.e., a plan adopted and implemented separately from the comprehensive plan such as a stormwater management plan and a trails and recreation plan, for example).

The actions described in the previous three bulleted items can also be applied to te following functional plans:

- Land use
- Transportation
- Streets and circulation
- Sidewalks
- Bicycle and pedestrian
- Parks, open space, recreation, trails
- Transit
- Health and social services
- Housing
- Economic development
- Schools and campuses
- Accessibility and universal design

THE THIRD POINT OF INTERVENTION: IMPLEMENTATION TOOLS

As is the case whenever a community revises its planning goals to address new concerns or new ways of thinking, achieving the goals related to health and physical activity in the comprehensive plan, function plans, or special area plans will require communities to rethink and retool their land development regulations (i.e., zoning and subdivision ordinances or unified ordinances) and other development regulations.

For example, a community could revise its ordinances to permit new urbanist or traditional neighborhood developments, either as an overlay, as a requirement in certain districts, or communitywide. Some communities will want to consider implementing a form-based code as an alternative to a conventional zoning ordinance. Such a code would help create neighborhoods and commercial districts without rigid constraints on land use. The emphasis in a form-based code on the scale and orientation of buildings relative to the street could also be used to create neighborhoods where walking is possible and pleasurable. Other tools that a health-savvy community might want to incorporate into its development regulations include the following, with illustrations:

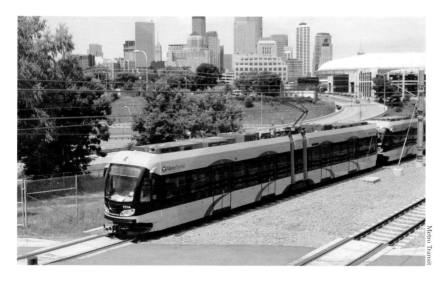

A study reported in the American Journal of Health Promotion *found that one-third of transit users are likely to walk more than 30 minutes a day. They would not otherwise get this physical activity without the trip to the transit stop (Besser and Dannenberg 2005). Shown here, the Hiawatha Light Rail in Minneapolis.*

Metro Transit

A study of trail use published in The Journal of Physical Activity and Health *found a significant correlation between people's use of trails and certain neighborhood characteristics, including income, neighborhood population density, education, percent of neighborhood in commercial use, vegetative health, area of land in parking, and mean length of street segments in access networks (Lindsay et al. 2006).*

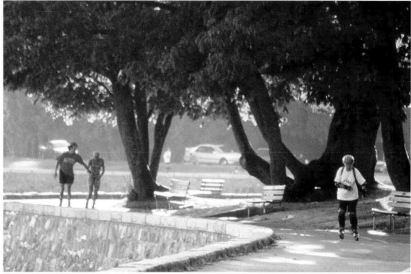

www.pedbikeimages.org/Dan Burden

Roundabout intersections, like this one in Gainesville, Florida, send a signal to drivers to reduce speed, making the streets safer for people on foot.

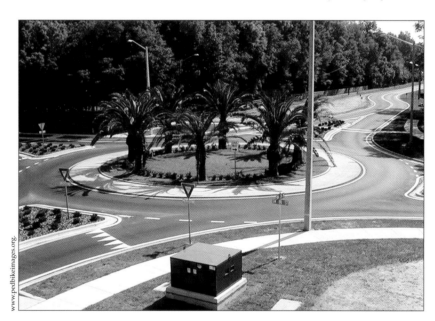

www.pedbikeimages.org

Bulbouts create shorter crossings for pedestrians while at the same time forcing automobiles to slow down as they enter the narrower space (Venice, Florida).

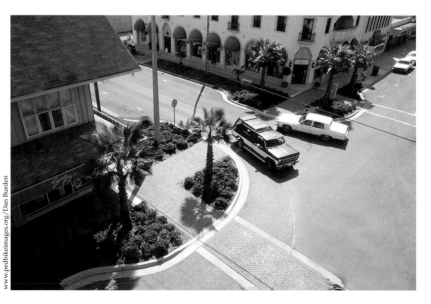

www.pedbikeimages.org/Dan Burden

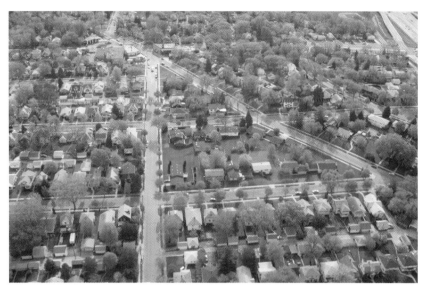

© Regents of the University of Minnesota. Used with the permission of the Metropolitan Design Center.)

Well-connected streets, with short blocks, choices of routes, and shorter trip distances affect people's decisions to walk, bike, or drive. A 2005 study in King County, Washington, showed a significant 14 percent increase in a person's decision to walk for each measured degree of increased street connectivity. Connectivity was measured using an index that combined the number of blocks, intersections, access points, cul-de-sacs, and linear feet of street in the study area (LUTAQH 2005).

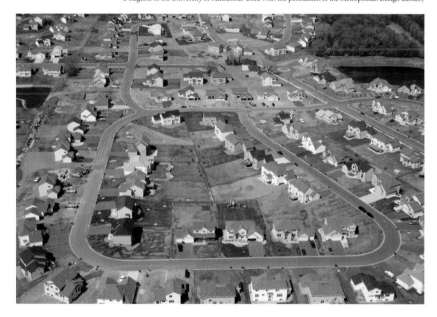

Smart Code Reforms of Zoning and Subdivision Regulations

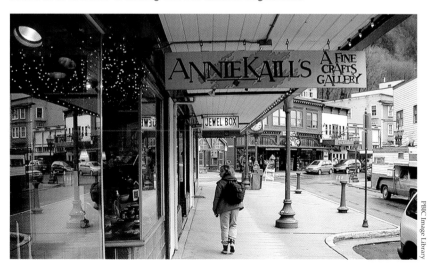

Streetscapes that feature a high level of building- and street-level detail—including ground-floor retail stores with ample windows—make the street a more interesting place from the standpoint of the pedestrian, thereby encouraging more walking (Frank and Engelke 2001).

Including landscaping in and around a parking lot not only creates a pleasant pedestrian environment but also reduces the amount of impervious surface coverage.

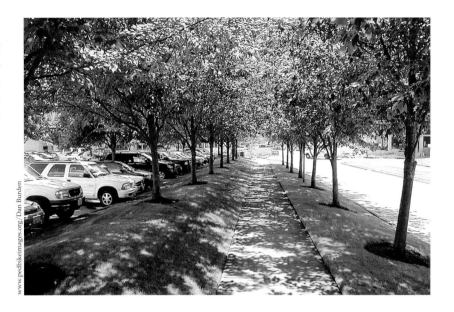

Belmont Dairy, an award-winning mixed-use development in Portland, contains 85 apartments and lofts as well as 26,000 square feet of retail space.

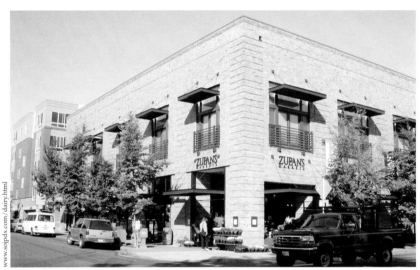

The recent development of Liberty on the Lake in Stillwater, Minnesota, is based on the new urbanist principles of pedestrianism and mixed use. The development offers traditional housing stock, narrower than normal streets, and sidewalks and footpaths that connect residences to the Rutherford Elementary School (pictured here).

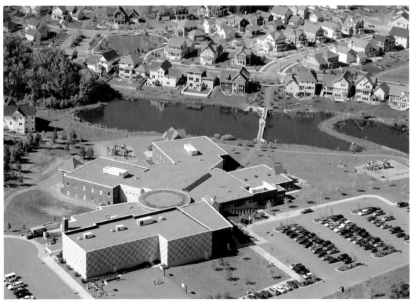

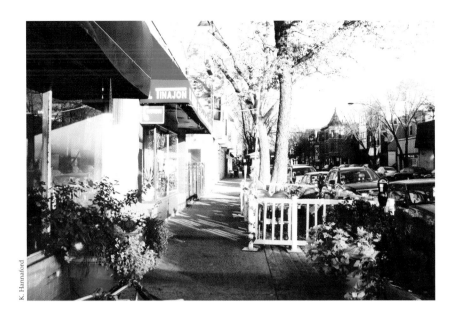

K. Hannaford

An urban village, such as the Roscoe Village neighborhood in Chicago, is characterized by a mix of housing types, neighborhood-serving retail stores, and services uses, such as groceries, hardware stores, dry cleaners, restaurants, and coffee shops. Commercial areas are built to a human scale, with ground-floor retail and apartments on the upper floors. Proponents of the urban village concept also call for a neighborhood school reachable by students on foot and for transit connections.

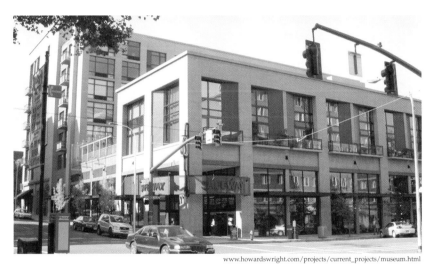

www.howardswright.com/projects/current_projects/museum.html

Museum Place in downtown Portland, Oregon, is a three-block project that includes a renovated YMCA, 500 rental housing units (including some set aside for low-income households), a grocery store, and ground-floor retail space.

Open Space and Recreation Facility Reforms

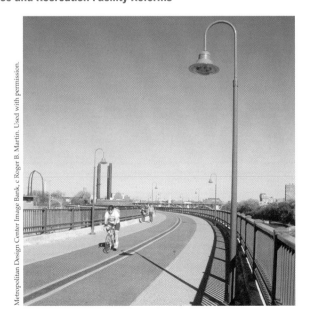

Metropolitan Design Center Image Bank, c Roger B. Martin. Used with permission.

People who live in low-income neighborhoods, receive health care at community clinics in their neighborhood, and reside near a trail are more likely to meet the recommended level of walking at least 30 minutes fives times per week compared to those who do not reside close to a trail (Pierce et al. 2006).

Active communities typically require developers to dedicate land or contribute cash in lieu of land to be used for parks, open space, and trails. Shown here, a park trail in Stapleton, a new urbanist development in Denver.

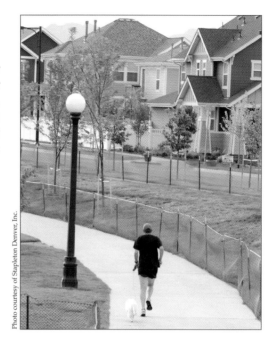

Mobility, Transportation, and Traffic Circulation Reforms

Requiring sidewalks to be a minimum of five feet wide (which is what is needed for two adults to walk side by side) on both sides of residential streets can encourage walking for transportation and recreation.

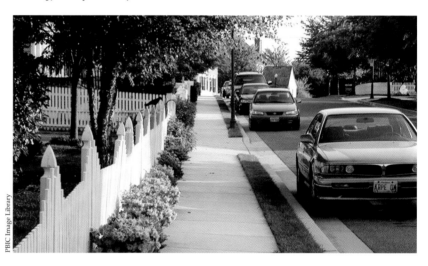

This crosswalk in San Diego features a pedestrian refuge island. It provides safe access across a busy arterial street to the neighborhood's only park.

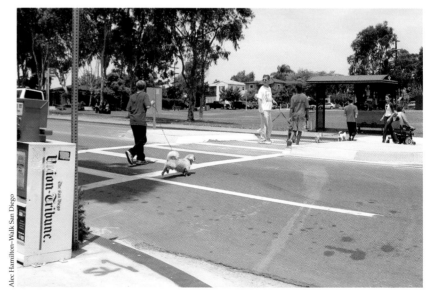

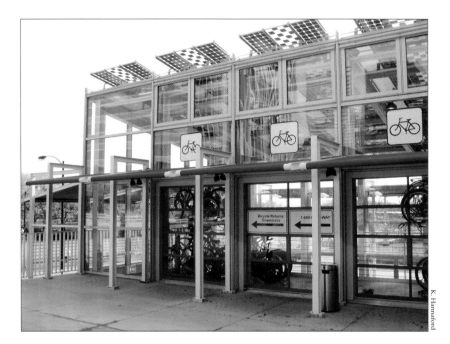

Designed to encourage bicycle commuting to downtown Chicago, Millennium Park's bicycle facility offers 300 secure indoor parking spaces for bikes, locker and shower facilities, bike repair services, and an outdoor café.

K. Hamaford

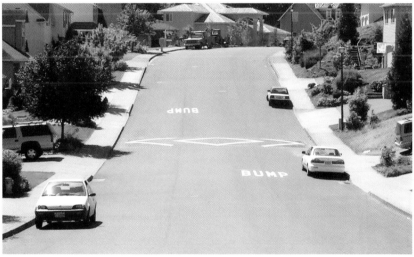

www.pedbikeimages.org/ITE Pedestrian Bicycle Council

According to a 2004 study by Morrison and Thomson reported in the Journal of Epidemiological Health, *the introduction of traffic calming devices, such as the speed bump shown here, are associated with increased pedestrian activity and improved physical health. It is important to note that a street narrower than the one depicted here could be equally or more effective in taming traffic, eliminating the need for speed bumps.*

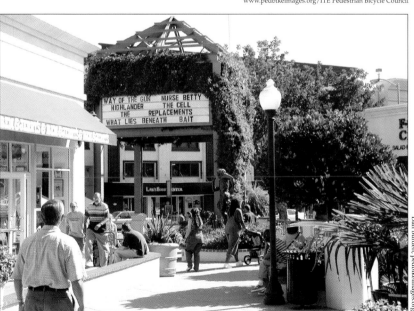

Dan Burden, pedbikeimages.org

Mission Plaza in San Luis Obispo, California, is a two-block pedestrian district with a large public plaza, seating areas, and pedestrian passageways between Mission Junipero Serra Del Tolosa and businesses on the opposite side of a San Luis Obispo Creek. The plaza has grown and evolved in three phases of development in the two decades.

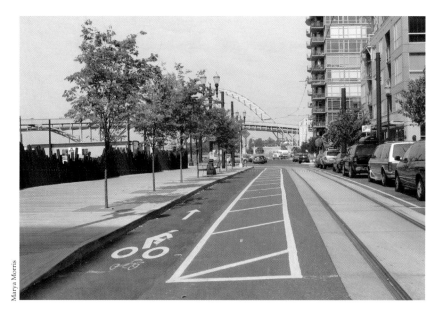

A "complete street," such as this block of 10th Street in the Pearl District in Portland, Oregon, is one designed and operated to enable safe access for pedestrians, bicyclists, transit users, and motorists.

Marya Morris

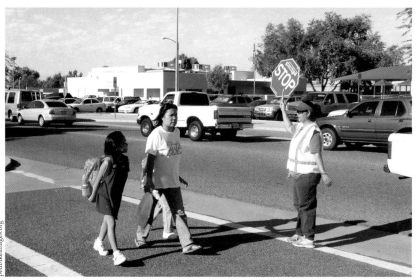

According to parents, school kids who see Safe Routes to School improvements being made in their neighborhoods (e.g., new sidewalks, crosswalks, traffic lights) are more likely to walk or bike to school because they perceive the route to be safe (Boarnet and Anderson 2005).

pedbikeimages.org

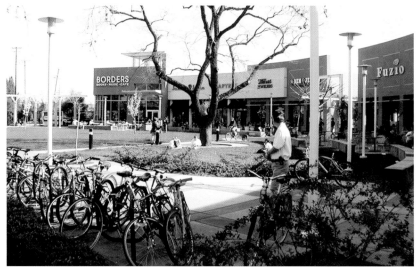

Ample lighting and bicycle parking make this shopping center a secure, inviting destination for bicyclists and pedestrians. Several studies have found a correlation between obesity and residents' perceptions that their neighborhood is unsafe because of crime and/or traffic (Burdette et al. 2006; Luming et al. 2006).

www.pedbikeimages.org/Dan Burden

Public Investment Reforms Should Address the Following Three Issues:

1. Directing public investment to targeted growth areas

2. Capital improvement programs

3. Equitable allocation of capital improvements spending on activity-friendly projects

THE FOURTH POINT OF INTERVENTION: SITE DESIGN AND DEVELOPMENT

Communities can make numerous improvements to the public realm and streetscapes to create attractive, safe places where people will want to walk, where it is safe for people of all ages and mobility levels to cross the street, where there is protection from inclement weather, where people feel protected from crime, and where there are opportunities for people to interact with one another. Planners can use a combination of design guidelines and urban design standards to work with developers to create such environments. Common tools include standards that: prohibit long, blank walls abutting sidewalks; require ground floors to have retail stores with windows; specify that buildings, especially those along transit routes and with heavy pedestrian traffic have awnings; require trees, landscaping, and street furniture to be added to the streetscape; and locate parking on the side or in the rear of commercial buildings. The planning department can negotiate with developers for these types of amenities or modifications to building and site design during the site plan review or design review process.

There are many intervention points in the site design and development stage that will support and protect public health, including the following:

1. Implement streetscape enhancements that include shade trees, awnings, art work, and pedestrian amenities, such as benches, to encourage people to be physically active.

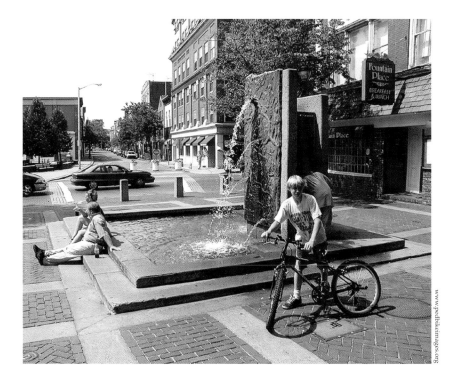

Fountains, plazas, and street art encourage people to use the street as a gathering place.

www.pedbikeimages.org

People to want to walk need interesting and aesthetically pleasing places to go. This shopping street integrates storefronts, street trees, and angled parking in an effective way.

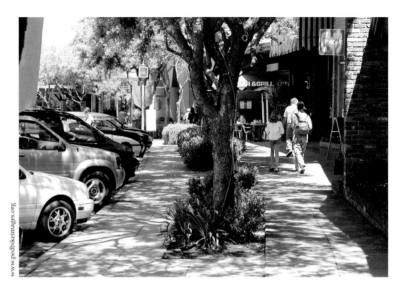

Uniform building orientation and setback standards can create a pedestrian-friendly environment that accommodates people on foot, transit users, and drivers.

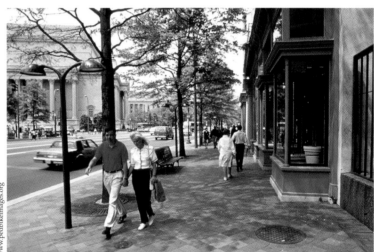

People may be moved to take the stairs if colorful materials, sculpture, and/or an open design are used, as was done in the Genetics, Developmental, and Behavioral Sciences Building at UC San Francisco, Mission Bay.

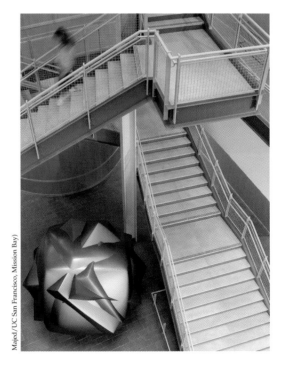

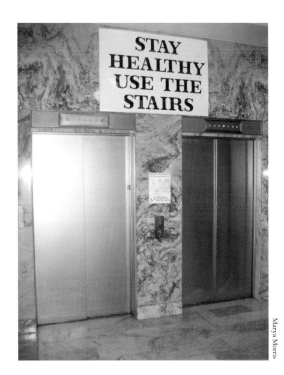

Marya Morris

Businesses can use motivational signage to increase the use of stairs.

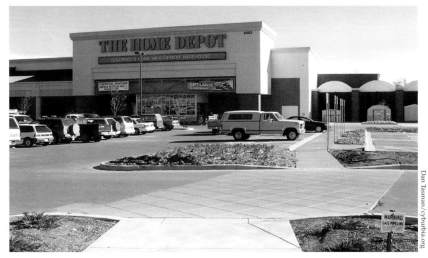

Dan Tasman/cyburbia.org

Using parking lot landscaping and variable pavement can make the trip for pedestrians from the street or transit stop safer and more welcoming

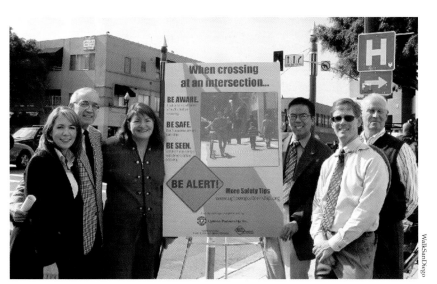

WalkSanDiego

WalkSanDiego worked with a neighborhood group and a local San Diego councilmember (Toni Atkins, in red) to launch a pedestrian safety campaign in the Hillcrest neighborhood, a favorite for walkers.

Shade trees, benches, traffic barriers, and inviting ground-floor retail space creates an ideal pedestrian environment on this street in Cambridge, Massachusetts.

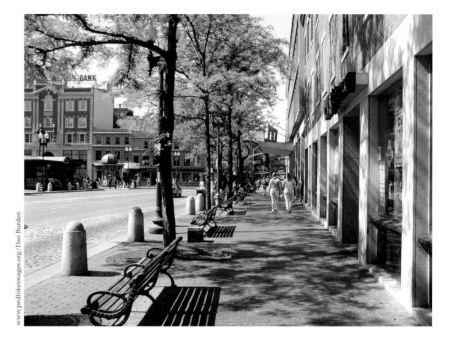

Trees not only provide shade and reduce temperatures in urban and suburban areas, they also provide a beautiful backdrop for pedestrian activity.

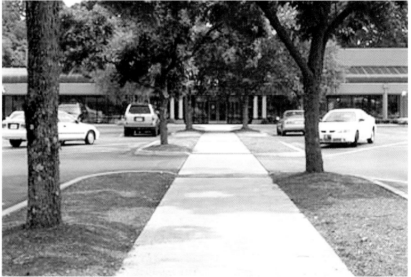

Courtesy of the Knoxville Knox County Metropolitan Planning Commission

THE FIFTH POINT OF INTERVENTION: PUBLIC FACILITY SITING AND CAPITAL SPENDING

Deciding where to locate and how to design public facilities (e.g., post offices, libraries, schools, and community centers) is important for communities serious about creating walkable environments. The most significant part of an individual's decision when making a trip on foot is having a purpose or a destination in mind. In addition to regular destinations like stores, schools, and workplaces, these public facilities serve as regular walking destinations and community gathering places. This is especially true for seniors and persons with a disability, who in general are more dependent on walking and transit for transportation than is the general population.

A recent and very popular approach to combating childhood inactivity and weight problems is to create safe routes for children to walk or bike to school. Researchers have found that children who live in neighborhoods with sidewalks are more likely to walk to school than those who live where there are no sidewalks (Ewing 2005). In Marin County, California, a safe-

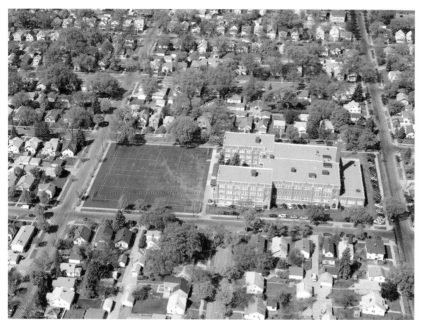

Until the 1950s, American schools were usually located within easy walking or biking distance of their students. Built in 1931 and still in use in the Standish neighborhood of Minneapolis, Minnesota, the Folwell Middle School exemplifies this type of pedestrian-accessible school.

© Regents of the University of Minnesota. Used with the permission of the Metropolitan Design Center.

routes-to-school program that included both street safety improvements and encouraged students to walk increased the number of students walking to school by 64 percent in two years (Staunton et al. 2003). See also Chapter 5 in this PAS Report for more on school siting and safety considerations.

CONCLUSION

It is important to note that the Five Strategic Points of Intervention framework essentially mirrors a typical planning process (i.e., one that begins with visioning and goal-setting sessions and ends with implementation of the plan through land-use regulations). In practice, users of this PAS Report may opt to begin with any of the five points, depending on what is happening in their jurisdiction and what is likely to have a positive impact on the public's health in the short or long term. We recognize, for example, functional plans are not necessarily prepared concurrently with a broader comprehensive planning effort. A trails and greenways plan may be undertaken separately, but in and of itself provides a key intervention point where health should be interjected. Further, a streetscape improvement plan in a specific neighborhood commercial core could provide an ideal opportunity for the community to consider measures to improve pedestrian safety and address crime.

The five points approach is intended to help planners and public health leaders and their staffs conceptualize how, when, and in what form health matters should be addressed in the planning process. There are no doubt other successful approaches used in communities that have already retooled their planning and land development regulations with the aim of creating healthier communities, including those described in Chapter 6 of this PAS report.

CHAPTER 4 LIST OF REFERENCES

[This List of References is supplemented by a Resource List at the end of this PAS Report.]

Boarnet, M. G., C. L. Anderson, et al. 2005. "Evaluation of the California Safe Routes to School Legislation: Urban Form Changes and Children's Active Transportation to School." *American Journal of Preventive Medicine* 28 (Supplement 2): 134–40.

Burdette, H. L., T.A. Wadden, and R.C. Whitaker. 2006. "Neighborhood Safety, Collective Efficacy, and Obesity in Women with Young Children." *Obesity* 14, no. 3: 518–25.

Frank, L., P. Engelke, T. Schmid, and R. Killingsworth. 2001. "The Built Environment and Human Activity Patterns: Exploring the Impacts of Urban Form on Public Health." *Journal of Planning Literature* 16, no. 2: 202–18.

Krizek, K. J., and P.J. Johnson. 2006. "Proximity to Trails and Retail: Effects on Urban Cycling and Walking." *Journal of the American Planning Association* 72, no. 1: 33-42.

Lindsey, G., Y. Han, J. Wilson, and J. Yang. 2006. "Neighborhood Correlates of Urban Trail Use." *Journal of Physical Activity and Health* 3 (Supplement 1): S139–57.

Lumeng, J. C., D. Appugliese, H. J. Cabral, R. H. Bradley, and B. Zuckerman. 2006. "Neighborhood Safety and Overweight Status in Children." *Archives of Pediatrics and Adolescent Medicine* 160, no. 1: 25–31.

Morrison, D. S., H. Thomson, et al. 2004. "Evaluation of the Health Effects of a Neighbourhood Traffic Calming Scheme." *Journal of Epidemiological Community Health* 58, no. 10: 837–40.

Pierce, J. R., A. V. Denison, A. A. Arif, and J. E. Rohrer. 2006. "Living Near a Trail Is Associated with Increased Odds of Walking among Patients Using Community Clinics." *Journal of Community Health* 31, no. 4: 289–302.

Puget Sound Regional Council and King County, Washington. 2004. *A Study of Land Use, Transportation, Air Quality and Health in King County, WA/LUTAQH*. Prepared by Lawrence Frank and Co., Inc.

CHAPTER 5

The ABCs of Creating and Preserving Accessible Community Schools

By Bruce Appleyard, AICP, and Timothy Torma

An accessible community school is one located in close proximity to the residences of its students and accessible by safe routes to those students who use means other than automobiles or buses to get to school. The problem in creating accessible community schools is the disconnect between school facility planning and other community planning functions. But even if a local planning commission or staff is not expressly authorized to influence school location and development policies, planners and school boards can take an active role in developing a common *community* agenda for issues related to the location and design of schools and in making sure schools are properly linked by safe routes for walkers and "rollers" (bicyclists, skateboarders, scooters, skaters, etc.).

This chapter will provide planners with a set of tools to constructively intervene and positively influence the planning of public schools so they are physically accessible to the communities they educate. It will also provide planners with the rationale, guidelines, and methods to create more schools that act as centers of their community and that can be easily reached via safe walking and /or rolling routes. To achieve this, planners need to be a part of the conversation and work with school districts and local officials to gain influence over school siting decisions so that those decisions are not made in a vacuum with no sense of their transportation or land-use impacts.

This chapter also provides a guide for planners on how to create conditions from a programmatic side that create safe access, thereby encouraging parents to allow their children to walk and bike to school, with a particular focus on the international movement known as Safe Routes to Schools (SR2S).

A BRIEF HISTORY OF U.S. SCHOOL AND NEIGHBORHOOD DESIGN: THE TREND FROM COMMUNITY SCHOOLS TO "BIGGER IS BETTER"

In the 1920s, architect Clarence Perry formalized the concept of building neighborhoods around schools in his writings on neighborhood unit. Perry articulated the six principles of the unit while participating as a member of the Community Center movement and the Regional Planning Association of New York, where he contributed to an extended process of regional planning for the New York Area between 1922 and 1929.

Perry's concept, influenced by British Town Designer Raymond Unwin, suggested that schools be placed in residential communities in such a way that a child would never have to cross a heavily trafficked street in order to get safely to school. His principles outlined the mixing of different types of

Figure 5-1. Illustration of Clarence Perry's neighborhood unit principles for schools.

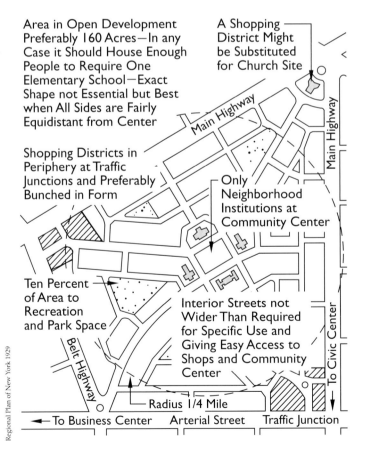

land uses, preserving open space, and having retail and other activities appropriately scaled to the community within which they are located. He also proposed a hierarchy of streets. If long blocks were used, pedestrian paths were to be constructed to offer shortcuts. He also made some of the earliest references to traffic calming, stating that if long, straight streets were used, measures to "compel cautious driving" should be employed.

Unfortunately, the publication of Perry's work coincided with the stock market crash in 1929. The U.S. housing market remained quiet for 15 years, throughout the Great Depression and World War II. Following WW II, many neighborhoods were developed around schools, but they often lacked key ingredients for making them truly walkable for many of the students. Most notably, neighborhood design moved into an era dominated by curvilinear and cul-de-sac street networks which often lacked sidewalks. In rapidly suburbanizing areas of California, for example, developers successfully argued before local government officials that no one wanted sidewalks because they were too urban, which allowed developers to sidestep the prevailing guidelines of the time. The developers' and the local officials' desire to save money by not building sidewalks no doubt aided their decision to build neighborhoods without sidewalks (Appleyard 1997).

Schools in the U.S. have grown steadily larger and larger since before WW II, both in terms of average number of students per school and in the size of school sites. The trend towards larger schools accelerated in the years immediately after the war.

According to the National Center for Educational Statistics (NCES) the number of public schools in the U.S. has decreased from approximately 247,000 in 1930 to 93,000 in 2002. Over the same time period, the student population has risen from 28 million to 53.5 million, and will grow to 60 million by 2030. As average school size has grown, the trend has been toward building consolidated "mega schools" at the edges of the communities they serve.

Why? In the middle of the twentieth century, a move arose to make schools larger and to build new ones rather than improve existing schools. A desire to improve educational outcomes partly explains the trend. James B. Conant, a Harvard-educated college administrator and scientist who studied American high schools argued for larger schools in his book, *The American High School Today* (1959), as a means of providing students with the most comprehensive high school education possible. His work is cited by those who advocated larger school districts and larger high schools as a means of providing a better education. Conant's notion of "too small" was a school with fewer than 100 students in 12th grade. Today, about half of U.S. secondary schools enroll more than 1,000 students. According to the U.S. Department of Education, approximately 70 percent of American high school students attend schools enrolling 1,000 or more students, and nearly 50 percent of high school students attend schools enrolling more than 1,500 students. Enrollments of 2,000 or more are common. Florida had the highest average secondary school size in the 2001–2002 school year at 1,565 students. Another rationale for both larger schools and larger school districts is the drive to achieve economies-of-scale.

CHANGING THE TREND IN SCHOOL SITING AND SIZE

Since the trend towards larger schools started, a large and diverse body of research has shown that smaller schools are better for students (see, generally, Irmsher 1997, for an excellent summary of the research on this subject). Smaller schools outperform large school across a wide array of indicators including academic performance, graduation rates, truancy, behavioral

Schools in the U.S. have grown steadily larger and larger since before WW II, both in terms of average number of students per school and in the size of school sites.

As planners we need to strike a balance that ensures that integration objectives are met at the same time we work toward creating and maintaining community accessible schools. Current trends, however, make it clear how difficult it will be to ensure that this balance occurs.

A study by the Civil Rights Project at Harvard University found that the nation's schools are becoming resegregated. According to the report, "A Multiracial Society with Segregated Schools: Are We Losing the Dream?" (www.civilrightsproject. harvard.edu/research/reseg03/resegregation03. php), the American South remains one of the most integrated parts of the country. One of the reasons Southern schools are managing to stay more integrated is that school districts are more likely to be countywide, encompassing both the urban core and suburban areas. These districts are more able to balance out segregated housing patterns. City school districts, on the other hand, don't have that option—desegregation across jurisdictional boundaries was struck down in a 1976 Supreme Court decision that kept Detroit from busing city children to suburban schools. The fragmentation of jurisdictions is one of the hallmarks of sprawl and has become a barrier to school desegregation. Some critics of small schools fear that they provide an opportunity for *de facto* segregation. They believe that students who are free to choose their small school will do so in a way that undermines the goal of social integration.

Rather than moving all students into larger schools, one approach to strike a balance between integration and transportation objectives is to maintain or build neighborhood-based elementary schools where significant portions of the students live, and then stagger grade levels. For example, make one elementary school the K-3, and the other a grade 4–5 (or 4–6). The students from one community would be able to walk to school, while the children from the other could bike or be bussed. Part of the way through, the community would switch who could walk and who would bike or be bussed. While not entirely ideal from the transportation objectives discussed in this chapter, more important community objectives of community integration and equality can be achieved. Finally, by having students travel into each other's neighborhoods, there is arguably a greater chance for more profound exchange across the social spectrum.

problems, student participation in school activities, parental involvement, student attitudes towards school, and others. As Mary Anne Raywid (1997), a researcher at Hofstra University put it, "There is enough evidence now of devastating effects of large size on substantial numbers of youngsters that it seems morally questionable not to act on this evidence."

So, if so much research suggests that larger schools are not good for students, why does the trend towards larger and larger schools continue? An important part of the answer lies in a variety of requirements and policies that influence school investments at the state and local levels. In some cases, these were intended specifically to facilitate bigger schools; in others, they have that effect as an unintended consequence. Together, they act as barriers to building or maintaining smaller schools that serve as centers of their community. To become effectively engaged in influencing school siting and size decisions, planners will need to become familiar with these barriers, find information that can help change the policies behind them, and help school districts adopt strategies to counteract them.

Minimum Acreage Standards

In the 1940s, the Council of Educational Facilities Planners International (CEFPI) first published guidelines suggesting minimum acreages for school sites. According to CEFPI, rather than being based on any formula or rationale, the guidelines were based on an informal survey of its membership at the time. It should be noted that CEFPI does not (and never has) set standards that schools must use. However, publication of guidelines in their materials was influential. Minimum acreage standards based on the CEFPI guidelines (or others using a similar formula) were subsequently adopted by many states as either requirements or recommendations to school boards. Today, many state and local policies and regulations still recommend *minimum* acreage standards for schools that are so large they often force schools to the fringe of urban areas where developable land is more plentiful.

The original CEFPI guidelines were as follows:

- Elementary Schools = 10 acres plus 1 acre for every 100 students
- Junior High/Middle Schools = 20 acres plus 1 acre for every 100 students
- Senior High Schools = 30 acres plus 1 acre for every 100 students

Using these guidelines, a 2,000-student high school would require *at least 50 acres of land*. In an effort to get a clearer picture of the role minimum acreage standards play in school siting, CEFPI researched state minimum acreage requirements in 2003 (available at: http://www.cefpi.org/pdf/state_guidelines.pdf). Their research showed that 27 states have some form of minimum site size policy or regulation for schools, with a wide range of specified sizes. Given the drawbacks of this approach, however, many states are rethinking such standards. In 2003, for example, South Carolina eliminated its minimum acreage requirements. In the early 1970s, Maryland decided not to establish any site size guidelines or standards.

Planners should be aware that a 2004 revision of CEFPI's influential *Guide for Planning Educational Facilities* no longer contains minimum acreage guidelines for school sites. Recognizing that a "one size fits all" approach is dated and can work counter to a variety of goals, the new *Guide* encourages communities to analyze their needs in order to make appropriate siting decisions. Many state and local school officials may not be aware of these changes to the CEFPI guidelines. Sharing this information with school officials may influence important investment decisions.

Policies that Favor New Construction over Renovation

In addition to the trend in school site size, another factor contributing to the decline of the accessible community school are state policies that favor the construction of new schools over the rehabilitation of older community-based schools. In 1952, Columbia University education professor Henry Linn, writing in *American School and University* (a trade magazine) suggested that if the cost of renovating a school was more than half what it cost to build new, school districts should forego renovation and build a new school. Though no clear rationale for this conclusion was (or has been since) provided, it has had a wide influence on school spending.

This influence is reflected in the fact that many state funding formulas authorize school renovations only when renovations will cost less than new construction (for example, when the cost of renovating a school is 75 percent or less of the cost of building a new school). Many states will not provide funding to school districts to rehabilitate older schools if the rehabilitation cost exceeds some preset percentage (such as 75 percent) of the cost of building a new school.

Renovation and/or expansion of existing schools rather than new construction can be cost-effective and a good decision for other reasons as well. Many older schools were built with much higher standards of architecture and construction. They also tend to be located within the communities they serve, making them more likely to be accessible via walking and rolling and to other members of the community. Older schools are also often a source of civic pride and serve as landmarks or anchors within their community. There is no "funding formula" that can adequately take many of these factors into account. Fortunately, there are resources for school boards and communities that want to make more deliberate decisions about older schools. In 2004, CEFPI published *A Primer for the Renovation/Rehabilitation of Older and Historic Schools,* which details many barriers and solutions to undertaking renovations or expansions of older schools (Gurwit 2004). The National Trust for Historic Preservation has also done extensive work documenting state and local policies that affect school renovation and provides case studies of successful renovations on its web site, www.nationaltrust.org/issues/schools/index.htm.

Lack of Coordination between School Facility Planning and Land-Use Planning

In many states, schools are exempt from local zoning regulations, while in others, local review is limited. Furthermore, in most states, school districts are not required to adhere to or even consult with the local comprehensive plan before making school siting decisions. Capital planning for schools is frequently not integrated with other local capital planning or economic development efforts. This lack of coordination is sometimes protected jealously by school boards who see coordination as a threat to their autonomy. Gerwin (2004) notes the difficulty planners may face:

> The attitude of many state school board associations is pretty well summed up by Ed Dunlap, who runs the North Carolina School Board Association. "Our position is very clear," he says. "It is the responsibility of the local board of education to make decisions about where schools are sited. Period."

Another factor contributing to the decline of the accessible community school are state policies that favor the construction of new schools over the rehabilitation of older community-based schools.

The trend towards large schools on the edges of the communities they serve has coincided with a steady rise in the number of students who receive transportation at public expense. This has also coincided with a precipitous drop in the numbers of students who walk and bike to school.

According to the National Center for Educational Statistics (NCES), 55.5 percent of all public primary and secondary school students were transported to school at public expense during the 2000-01 school year (http://nces.ed.gov/programs/digest/d03/tables/dt167.asp). In terms of raw numbers, that represents more than 24 million kids. The cost of transporting these students exceeded $14 billion in 2000–01.

The NCES historical data on student transportation reveal some long-term trends with implications for school systems, school budgets, student health, and community planning.

- The percentage of students transported at public expense rose steadily from 8.9 percent in 1929 to more than 60 percent in the mid-1980s. At that point, the trend leveled and began a slow decline to the 55.5 percent rate of 2000–01. One explanation for the reversal in the 1990s is the rise in the number of parents who drive kids to school and the number of students who drive themselves to school. Another is that some court-ordered busing programs to implement desegregation have lapsed.

- The cost per student for bus transportation has risen steadily. In constant-dollar terms, it has risen from a low of $226 per student transported in 1947–48 to the 2000–2001 level of $575.

- In South Carolina, for just one example of state spending on busing, the state education department buys more than 12 million gallons of diesel fuel each year for its 5,000 buses. Each time the fuel rate goes up a penny, it costs the state about $120,000. When gas prices rise, as they did in 2005 and 2006, the agency almost certainly will bust its budget and have to ask the governor and lawmakers for help.

Beyond these raw numbers and costs, the issue of school busing trends, impacts, and more has received remarkably little research in the last 40 years. Given the impact that busing has on overall education budgets and how families and students relate to their schools, this area is ripe for closer scrutiny. (See Howley 2000 for an examination of this finding and a suggested research agenda.) ▪

Some places are proactively seeking to address this issue. For example, Florida law requires that local governments and school boards enter into interlocal agreements that address school siting, enrollment forecasting, school capacity, infrastructure, colocation, and joint use of civic and school facilities, sharing of development and school construction information, and dispute resolution (www.dca.state.fl.us/fdcp/DCP/SchoolPlanning/school_planning.htm).

Separation of School Siting Decisions from Long-Term Transportation Costs

Bus transportation of students is often paid largely by the state from a different funding stream than that used for capital improvements. Anecdotal evidence suggests little incentive exists for school siting decisions to take long-term transportation costs into account. Money that will be spent— potentially for decades to come—on transporting students to far-flung "cheaper" sites might be better used to select a site with higher upfront costs closer to the students it serves.

Deferred Maintenance

Many states support spending on new construction, but few support spending on routine maintenance (Lawrence 2003). Money for repairs is rarely included in school operating budgets, so other sources to fund such projects must be identified. Finding such funding is usually difficult at best. Maintenance is often deferred in favor of more urgent expenditures or those related more directly to education. Over time, this can lead to school buildings that need substantial investment simply to remain safe and functional. If the building requires extensive repairs or renovation, deferred maintenance may even lead to its closure, particularly in states that set requirements the existing school or site can't meet.

In addition to the many negative outcomes associated with deferred maintenance for the building and students, it can also act as yet another factor favoring construction of large new schools rather than investing in existing facilities. Each year of deferred maintenance makes the proposition of modernizing and improving a school building more daunting and more expensive. Patterns of deferred maintenance can lead to closure of older schools and feed the trend of school sprawl.

Some states have actively addressed this issue. The Aging School Program in Maryland provides State funds to all school systems to improve or maintain their aging school buildings. These funds can be used for capital improvements, repairs, and deferred maintenance work at existing public school buildings (see www.pscp.state.md.us/Programs/ASP/ADMINPROCASP percent202002.doc).

In Massachusetts, the School Building Assistance Program provides "incentive percentage points" for school renovation/reuse proposals. Such points increase the percentage of funding the state will provide for renovations and reuse projects. New school construction does not receive points (see www.mass.gov/msba/). Massachusetts also has funding conditions that make it difficult to get state funding for new school construction if a school has been closed in the jurisdiction in recent years (see www.doe.mass.edu/lawsregs/603cmr38.html?section=03). This provision acts as an incentive not to defer maintenance and favors upgrading existing facilities rather than closing them and building new.

Biased Funding Rules

A major roadblock to renovation is state funding policy that provides money for new school construction but not for restoration projects. In the mid-1990s, the Pittsburgh school board announced plans to replace two, small, wood-framed school buildings with one large addition to the local high school. When a neighborhood group, Save Our Schools, lobbied the school board to save the historic structures, they discovered the state would not provide money for renovations on two-story, wood-frame schools and would not reimburse districts for renovations that cost more than 60 percent of what it would cost to replace the school. The Pittsburgh History and Landmarks Foundation did a study showing that, out of 6,200 fire incidents recorded by the U.S. Fire Administration between 1991 and 1995, there was no correlation of the construction types and the number of injuries sustained. This convinced the Pennsylvania legislature to change their funding policy, and thus historic wood frame schools can be rehabilitated, as long as fire safety regulations can be met.

A PLANNER'S ROLE IN CREATING ACCESSIBLE COMMUNITY SCHOOLS

In many states, local planning agencies and planning commissions or boards have no authority to review school siting and design decisions even on an advisory basis. What is more, most school districts are not bound by local zoning or even environmental review. Nevertheless, planners can still take an active role in developing a common community agenda between school districts and local governments so that schools can fit within the community's comprehensive plans, goals and objectives.

First, planners must be able to explain the numerous advantages of accessible neighborhood schools. The section immediately below offers some talking points for planners first engaging in the school planning process. Second, planners, in a way similar to the one described in the previous chapter, need to understand the process of school siting and funding so as to find the most strategic points of intervention to encourage decision makers to put accessible community schools on an even playing field with large schools on the edge of communities and neighborhoods. Knowing the barriers (described above) to accessible community schools and knowing the possible points of intervention may give land-use planners a greater voice than they have ever had in school siting and shaping overall community development to achieve active living goals for young people and their parents. The subsections following a discussion of talking points describe briefly the school planning process and the possible points of intervention for planners. Finally, more is discussed about the possible role planners can play in transportation planning as it relates to schools, with special emphasis given to the Safe Routes to Schools Program (SR2S).

Talking Points

Below are some talking points to help planners discuss with school administrators, board members, parents, and the public the implications and opportunities related to siting schools. These points can help explain why it is important to have accessible community schools and educate the officials and the public about the relationship between community design and healthy physical activity, as well as the impact on health of traffic congestion, unsafe streets, and poor air quality.

- Obesity and diabetes rates in children are skyrocketing due in part to the lack of regular physical activity. Accessible schools give children an opportunity to make physical activity (i.e., walking or bicycling to school) part of their daily routine.

- Accessible neighborhood schools can give children and parents options about how to travel to school. These options can provide more independence for parents and children and more safety and activity for children.

- Neighborhood traffic that children may encounter on their route to school can be easier to tame and require less public investment for a community

Obesity and diabetes rates in children are skyrocketing due in part to the lack of regular physical activity. Accessible schools give children an opportunity to make physical activity (i.e., walking or bicycling to school) part of their daily routine.

than what would be required to create safe routes to larger schools on the urban fringe.

Accessible neighborhood schools give children an opportunity to make physical activity (i.e., walking or bicycling to school) part of their daily routine.

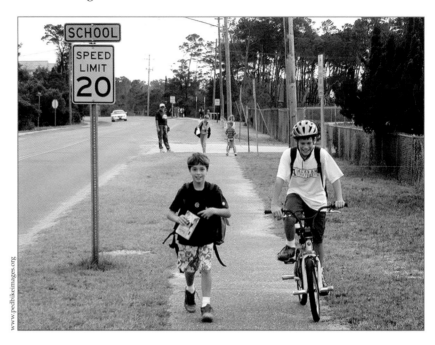

www.pedbikeimages.org

- Parents driving their children to school represent a significant number of car trips, which cause traffic congestion and affect air quality on the school grounds. While busing children to school does decrease the number of auto trips to and from schools, buses also contribute to traffic congestion and poor air quality. An EPA study of two high schools in Gainesville, Florida, suggested that neighborhood schools could generate 13 percent more walking or biking trips and 15 percent fewer auto emissions than schools built outside a community (EPA 2004).

It's 11 am outside this middle school (above), why would teachers, parents, and students at this school have cause for concern about traffic congestion and poor air quality on school grounds? Here's why (below): A twice daily traffic jam of idling cars waiting to pick up kids whose parents have no choice but to drive them to school.

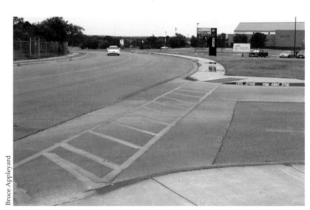

Bruce Appleyard

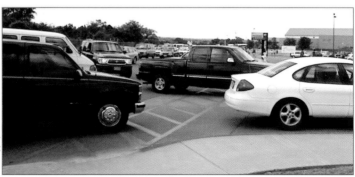

Bruce Appleyard

- When siting a new school, the school district and other local government bodies should consider the full costs of where a school is located on the community's entire budget, including family auto-operating expenses and costs of extending water and sewer infrastructure and roads.

- State funding for school busing has grown scarce, and local governments are struggling more and more to secure them. Second, with oil prices likely to continue to rise, the need to consider the full cost of transportation on the family budget as well as the locality's is necessary.

- An SR2S program can help institute the practice of children getting to school on their own. (SR2S principles and programs are described in greater detail below.)

- Schools not only can support the academic needs but can also address the social, educational, recreational, and personal needs of the members of the broader community. In particular, schools can provide:

  - public meeting space for neighborhoods meetings;

  - playground, exercise, and ballplaying facilities for community recreation and health; and

  - space for adult learning.

- Addressing parents' concerns about the safety of their children from an encounter with a dangerous stranger is requires the utmost care and thoughtfulness on the planner's part. In the initial conversation about this issue, leave out any statistics. The statistical probabilities should not be depended upon to make your points; to a parent, the specter of losing a child to a stranger is so terrible that relying on the statistics will appear callous. Principals and school officials will also be sensitive to the feelings of the parents. In fact, it is perhaps better to wait until someone asks about the statistical realities before you bring them up. And here is what you can say: According to Frank Furedi's book, *The Culture of Fear,*

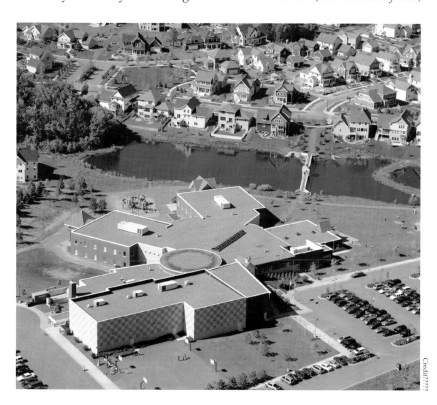

Liberty on the Lake in Stillwater, Minnesota, is New Urbanist development that offers traditional housing stock, narrow streets, sidewalks, and footpaths that connect students to the Rutherford Elementary School.

All school districts, even those with declining enrollment, develop their facility needs for every 10- to 20-year period and involve the local government and the public.

while the number of childhood abductions hasn't changed, the perceptions are that they have increased. The U.S. Department of Justice has also reported a fairly sharp decrease in the number of crimes against children ages 12–15 (specifically, a 27 percent decrease from 1994 to 1997) that parallels a decrease in victimization of adults in the same time frame (see www.unh.edu/ccrc/factsheet.html#1). Instead of discussing statistics, highlight how a community accessible school can offer can offer a safer street environment overall in the following ways:

- It allows neighbors and other parents to live along the route to school, providing "eyes on the street."

- By being close to the school, parents are better able to be "block parents" and to participate in running "walking school buses" (discussed below).

- Neighbors are better able to notice strangers and odd behavior on their street. A major concern surrounding child abduction is that a perpetrator will easily drive away with a child. In schools on the community fringe, this is likely to be more easily accomplished.

School Facility Planning and Enrollment Forecasting

For planners to have influence on school siting decisions, they must become familiar with a number of important aspects of the process. These include the preparation of a school facilities plan, the forecasting of enrollment and demographic trends, the formation of school siting advisory committees, and the funding sources and budgeting methods of the district.

In most states, a school facilities master plan is required in fast-growing school districts. These plans contain information about school closure, repair, expansion, modernization, renovation, and new construction. They are often driven by enrollment and demographic forecasts, so it is important to conduct these forecasts properly (see below).

One recommendation is that all school districts, even those with declining enrollment, develop their facility needs for every 10- to 20-year period and that they involve the local government and the public. Regular updates allow the school districts to communicate their vision to the public and the localities, and to respond to changes in the community.

Enrollment and demographic forecasts reveal how many families are moving in and out of the school district, rates of new home construction and existing housing sales, and birth rates.

In reviewing these documents and/or selecting sites for new schools, planners should consider the following:

- Whether the district's school plans are compatible with the community's comprehensive plan

- The proximity of the student population that will be served to the proposed new school

- How opportunities for students to walk or bike to school can be maximized

- The potential for new partnerships between the school, the neighborhood, and the community, such as using the school for communitywide events in after school hours and on weekends and holidays

- The relationship between the site and other public facilities, such as water, sewer, transit service, and roads

- The impact of new school construction on older, existing schools in the community

School District Construction Advisory Committees

Planners should make a concerted effort to get a professional planner or a planning commissioner represented on the construction advisory committee to ensure that planned school investment and siting decisions are informed and ideally influenced by other community goals, such as creating neighborhoods where schools are the center of the community. If the school planning board does not have a formal review body, a planner should consider providing an informal, advisory review of the school facility plan or providing input on a particular school project. A school district might appreciate the feedback, and it would strengthen channels of communication between school and planning staff to the point where school districts would start thinking about the broader, communitywide implications of their school siting decisions.

School Financing and Budgeting

Although formulas vary widely from state to state, most funding for school construction comes from local property tax revenue and state income revenue. In addition, many school districts have the power to raise money for school construction through bonds.

Local planning departments and planning commissions rarely have any formal role in reviewing the school district's capital budget. Rather, the school budget is formally presented to the local governing body for approval (e.g., the county board of supervisors or the city council).

In a best case scenario, the school board's decisions on school siting and capital investments would take into account community goals outside the scope of their typical decision criteria. These include siting schools in a manner that some or all children can walk or bike to school, encouraging rehabilitation of older school buildings, and establishing schools as a community anchor.

Planners should review how school investment decisions are made in their jurisdiction. In many communities, the planning commission prepares, or provides comments on, the local capital improvement plan. This is an opportune time for planners to raise questions about the relationship between your community's capital improvement plan and the school district's capital investment or construction plans.

Never underestimate the fiscal argument for building accessible community schools. When education bonds are on the ballot, partnerships that integrate community resources and services with a school's educational program can strengthen support from citizens, even those with no school-age children. Furthermore, planners should work with school districts and other groups in the area to put together school proposals that also meet broader community needs, providing facilities that can be used by all citizens (e.g. athletic fields, libraries, theaters). Find out what state and local policies or rules drive school investment decisions in your town. Some "rules" are actually just policies and are more flexible than most people realize. For example, a community in a state with minimum acreage standards may be able to get a waiver for a smaller school site.

Can't Get a Seat at the School Planning Table? Try Offering Carrots

In jurisdictions where local government has limited or no official role in the school planning process, it may take a lot of creativity and hard work to get a seat at the table. Of course, a little money never hurts either.

The Orange County Commission in North Carolina was looking for a creative way of linking school planning to other community goals. The commission proposed offering "bonus funds" to the school board for school construction if other community goals are met. Under this approach, the

A NOTE ABOUT SCHOOL ENROLLMENT AND DEMOGRAPHIC FORECASTS

Planners need to determine if they are using the same demographic data as are schools when making projections.

Good school enrollment forecasts incorporate land-use information, including knowledge about all the new subdivision plans at all the different stages, sketch, preliminary, and final approval. This is not always easy, given the divide between planning departments and school districts. It is recommended that the person in charge of forecasting school size request notification by the local planning department, responsible for the development review of new subdivisions.

Some caution should be exercised when basing forecasts on housing trends because they have been shown to overstate the projection of school enrollment, due in part to shrinking family size.

According to enrollment forecasting experts, most uncertainty and error occurs when trying to estimate how many children are in the "birth to kindergarten" age range.

Recognize an increase in enrollment in private schools often occurs when the economy is strong, and vice versa.

county commission awarded Chapel Hill-Carrboro City Schools (CHCCS) bonus funds for incorporating specific smart growth strategies in the construction of its third high school.

The bonus funds approved by the county commissioners provided the school district with an additional $1.9 million for the school, pending the implementation of smart growth measures, such as compact design, increased bus use, reduced parking, and sufficient sidewalks and paths to encourage student walking and biking. In June 2004, the school board agreed to design the new school with bike lanes and racks, but with parking spots for only 22 percent of the expected 800 students. The school board will receive an additional $300,000 if it agrees to a set of transportation initiatives laid out by the commission, including shuttles, park-and-ride shelters, and sidewalk improvements.

In this instance, the school's location was selected before the school board developed its smart growth goals, so siting was not part of the smart growth criteria. However, site selection is a critical component in determining how a school relates to the community it serves. Planners and local government officials who are considering use of a similar approach should strive to have it in place before decisions about the site of proposed schools are made. This approach comes with a price tag, but then again, the entire community will pay for poor school siting decisions for generations.

Transportation: Safe School Access, Neighborhood Traffic Management, and Safe Routes to Schools

Planners have several key points of intervention where they can provide input on school districts' transportation-related policies and programs. These actions can apply to either existing community schools or newly built schools, and can provide a basis for a comprehensive SR2S program.

At the overall capital facilities planning level, planners can be advocates for rehabilitating and modernizing older neighborhood-centered school facilities as the first option to consider prior to forging ahead with siting a new school that may serve some or most of the same students who attend the older school.

Where a new school is determined to be necessary, planners can advocate for siting the facility as close as possible to students' homes and neighborhoods. For new and existing schools, planners can work with traffic engineers to prepare a neighborhood traffic management plan to facilitate student pick-up and drop-off, so as to make safe the routes for children to walk

For both new schools and neighborhood schools, planners—working with traffic engineers and school representatives—can examine the site and community design to determine if there are safe routes linking the school to the community. Such an examination would determine such things as:

- where students, faculty, and staff live and how they arrive at school each day;

- the adequacy of existing or planned walking/ bicycling facilities (walkways, crosswalks and bike lanes, bike racks, etc.) not only at the site, but also connecting into adjoining neighborhoods; and

- the placement and timing of construction for pedestrian and bicycle facilities (i.e., will they be built by the time a new school opens).

Assuming the school can be placed in a location that is in close proximity to the community, a comprehensive SR2S program can make sure that the school becomes an enduring accessible community school. The next section describes SR2S programs in more detail.

SAFE ROUTES TO SCHOOL PROGRAMS

Following examples from Europe and Canada (see sidebar), the SR2S movement in the U.S. is an attempt to remove or redress the physical and psychological barriers to walking and biking between home and school. The potential payoffs associated with fostering healthier lifestyles are huge. Already, obesity among children in the U.S. has reached epidemic proportions according to the Centers for Disease Control and Prevention, in large part attributable to lower levels of physical activity. The obesity rate for children has tripled over the past two decades, a trend partially attributable to the inadequate infrastructure to support routine walking and biking. In addition, asthma rates have increased 160 percent in the past 15 years due in part to increased exposure to exhaust from automobiles.

SR2S programs can help battle child pedestrian injuries and fatalities which, according to the National Safe Kids Campaign, are the second leading cause of unintentional injury-related death among children ages 5 to 14 years old, in spite of the aforementioned downward trend of walking trips.

SR2S is an unusual approach to managing transportation. First, it has support from multiple constituencies (transportation, smart growth, public health and safety advocates, parents, teachers, and children) and has manifested itself in a variety of forms. Second, SR2S programs have gained strength from the local and grassroots level, resonating with the desire to recapture the cherished and independent expression of our childhood—the walk/bike to school. And third, where most other transportation strategies focus primarily on marketing and promotion (e.g., campaigns promoting carpooling and/or riding transit), SR2S puts an equal or greater emphasis on the provision of infrastructure improvements for walking and biking. Fueling the interest in SR2S is the increasing recognition of the physical disconnect between our schools and homes due to distance and the often frustrating lack of adequate infrastructure.

In concept, SR2S programs call for a focus on outcomes more than activities. The goal is to improve the health and well-being of our children by ensuring that most children can and do walk or bike to school most of the time. This vision for our schools can only be realized by:

- locating schools in close proximity to the children who attend them;
- providing good facilities for walking and biking to school;
- reducing the threats to health and safety posed by motor vehicles, pollution, and crime; and
- fostering a cultural shift that accords high value and broad responsibility for the realization of this goal.

SR2S programs rely on four primary elements, referred to as the Four Es: Engineering, Education, Encouragement, and Enforcement.

Engineering

Engineering involves more than just the provision of physical infrastructure, such as walkways, bike lanes, and crosswalks; it also includes strategic thinking about how these facilities are used. For example, engineers need to consider such things as closing gaps in discontinuous sidewalks and designating "bicycle boulevards," traffic-calmed routes to school that provide adequate space for cyclists and the fewest possible conflict points with automobiles.

Furthermore, engineering includes the use of low-cost, effective measures, such as trimming shrubs that limit sight distance and encroach into walkways, and installing higher visibility signs and pavement markings.

THE ORIGINS OF THE SAFE ROUTES TO SCHOOL MOVEMENT

In the mid-1970s, Denmark was cited as having the worst child pedestrian accident rate in Europe. This prompted the city of Odense to pioneer a pilot program to identify specific road dangers that students might face on their trip to school. They proceeded to create a network of traffic-free pedestrian and bicycle paths, established slow-speed areas for certain roads, and complemented these with traffic calming measures. In 10 years, child pedestrian and cyclist casualties fell by more than 80 percent. Soon after, Denmark established what is considered the longest standing national program, which has now been implemented in 65 localities nationwide.

In Great Britain, a group called Sustrans initiated 10 Safe Routes to Schools pilot projects in 1995. Bike lanes, traffic calming, and raised crossings cut traffic speed considerably. Two years into the initiative, bike use tripled. In the reduced-speed zones, child pedestrian casualties fell a dramatic 70 percent and cycling casualties by 28 percent.

Two Canadian programs were developed in the late nineties, borrowing from the success of the European examples. "Go for the Green in Toronto" and "Way to Go" in British Columbia both focus on creating safer routes near schools and initiating events and contests to encourage more children to walk and bike.

One of the earliest Safe Routes to School programs in the U.S. was started in New York City, in 1997, when Transportation Alternatives, a nonprofit public interest organization, and The Bronx Borough President's Office, created The Bronx Safe Routes to School program to work with parents, principals, teachers, community leaders, and city agencies to create pedestrian improvements around 38 elementary schools.

More recently, the Surface Transportation Policy Project and Transportation Alternatives produced a report on SR2S programs that provides a useful overview on the development of this movement in the U.S. The report is available at www.transact.org/report.asp?id=49.

The development of regular events throughout the year provides for program continuity. For example, some groups designate all Wednesdays as "Walking Wednesdays" (or Tuesdays, or . . .), so that every week a planned activity promotes walking and bicycling.

Education

The education component of SR2S aims to provide lifelong traffic safety skills to children, and their parents, about walking, bicycling and driving. These programs can be designed as a regular part of the school curriculum, or as part of an extra-curricular program. Education can also cover the health and environmental benefits of safe routes to school. The Pedestrian and Bicycle Information Center (www.pedbikeinfo.org) has excellent educational resources pertinent to many aspects of this PAS Report and, in particular, a web site devoted specifically to SR2S programs (www.walktoschool-usa.org).

Encouragement

The main objectives of the encouragement component within an SR2S program are to increase public awareness and support for SR2S goals and to promote changes in behavior. Activities may include: media and social marketing campaigns; special events such as a Walk to School Day and in-classroom contests; presentations to school and community groups, including elected officials; and SR2S program promotions. Encouragement programs might also include surveys of current practices and attitudes, such as how kids currently get to and from school, and what kinds of concerns parents have about allowing their children to walk or bike.

Enforcement

The primary objective of a SR2S program regarding enforcement is to reduce threats to the health and safety of children associated with the careless operation of motor vehicle, as well as other kinds of criminal behavior, including child abduction (often referred to as Stranger Danger). Activities include working with police, crossing guards, parents, and volunteers, such as block parents, to increase adherence to traffic laws by pedestrians and bicyclists as well as drivers, and to give appropriate attention to general crime prevention. Engaging community members in the street environment and providing more "eyes on the street" will help ensure that they endure as safe environments.

How Planners Can Help Get Safe Routes to School Programs Off and Running

While SR2S programs can take many forms, four activities are particularly effective in getting a program started:

1. The creation of a SR2S Team representing the many stakeholders in the community. The membership should include children, parents, and teachers, as well as other community residents, business owners in the school neighborhood, police, and public works engineers.

2. A well-planned kickoff event can generate excitement and cultivate a sense of community ownership that will carry the program forward. International Walk to School Day, which is usually in the first part of October, presents an ideal event to rally around.

3. The development of regular events throughout the year provides for program continuity. For example, some groups designate all Wednesdays as "Walking Wednesdays" (or Tuesdays, or . . .), so that every week a planned activity promotes walking and bicycling.

4. The convening of annual community workshops permits the SR2S Team to solicit additional input and disseminate information about the program

Conducting two surveys early in the process is a good idea. Students can be surveyed to determine how they get to school while parents' attitudes are measured to identify obstacles and opportunities for changing behavior.

As a starting point for planning for SR2S infrastructure, a careful analysis of the corridors leading to schools needs to be conducted during school arrival and dismissal times to observe students and traffic and to inventory problems.

STATE POLICIES, LAWS, AND REGULATIONS TO HELP CREATE ACCESSIBLE COMMUNITY SCHOOLS

As more states realize the benefits of accessible community schools, many are revising old regulations, passing new laws, or implementing innovative policies to encourage these facilities. Nine examples of state policies, laws, and regulations that can support community-centered schools are described briefly here. If your state does not use these policies, laws, or regulations, perhaps it is time to start a campaign for instituting some of them.

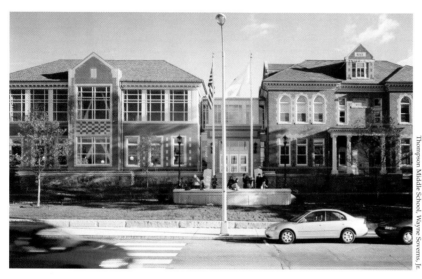

A $19 million bond issue that voters approved in 1999 financed the renovation and expansion of the historic Thompson Middle School in Newport, Rhode Island. Located just off Newport's Main Street downtown, the school serves as a community center and is well within walking distance for students and local residents who use the school for civic events after school hours.

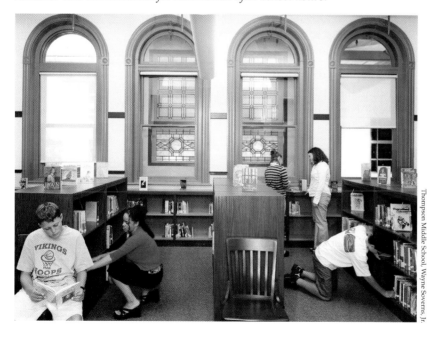

1. *Encourage school renovation by revising financing formulas.* The Ohio School Facilities Commission now allows waivers to its "2/3 rule." This rule withheld state funds for projects in which school renovation costs exceed two-thirds of the cost of new school construction. In such cases, school boards were forced to build new or forfeit the state money. School districts may now seek waivers to the "2/3 rule" when historic schools or "other good cause[s]" are involved. Allowing a waiver is helpful, but eliminating such rules altogether should be considered. The National Trust for Historic Preservation has urged states to eliminate these funding policies because they make it difficult for communities to maintain existing schools and bring them up to state-of-the-art standards, even when doing so costs less than building new.

2. *Require information sharing and coordinated planning between school districts and local planning agencies.* Under Florida's growth management strategy, local governments and district school boards must enter into interlocal agreements to share information regarding school planning and land development, and must collaborate in making school and land-use decisions. Failure to enter into the interlocal agreement subjects both the local governments and district school boards to financial sanctions.

3. *Use schools to promote smart growth development and redevelopment.* The Schools Renaissance Zone Program in New Jersey is based on the concept that new school facilities can serve as catalysts for redevelopment and investment. The SRZ program expands the focus from the school facility and focuses on needed improvements in the neighborhoods surrounding the schools. The program's emphasis is on the coordination of state assistance through a "zone team" comprised of members of state departments and agencies. Examples of neighborhood redevelopment might include construction of new or rehabilitated residential units, commercial development, streetscape improvements, and investment in community recreational, cultural assets, and open space. (For more on New Jersey, see http://www.njscc.com/CommunitySchools/AboutSchoolRenaissanceZones/RolesOfPartners/RolesOfPartners.asp.)

4. *Direct state funds to schools in existing communities.* The Maryland Public School Construction Program recommends that schools be located in developed areas, or in designated growth areas, be served by existing infrastructure, and not be developed in previously undeveloped areas. (For more on the Maryland program, see http://www.pscp.state.md.us/.)

5. *Set aside funds for aging schools.* The Aging School Program (ASP) in Maryland provides state funds to all school systems in the state to address the needs of their aging school buildings. These funds may be utilized for capital improvements, repairs, and deferred maintenance work at existing public school buildings and other sites serving students. (See www.pscp.state.md.us/Programs/ASP/ADMINPROCASP percent202002.doc.)

6. *Reduce or eliminate acreage standards for schools.* Size and location matter when creating accessible community schools. Currently, 27 states have some type of minimum acreage standard. However, given the drawbacks discussed elsewhere in this chapter, many states are rethinking this approach. In 2003, South Carolina eliminated its minimum acreage requirements. Maryland's decision to abandon acreage requirements dates to the 1970s, when the state recognized that acreage standards would force older cities like Baltimore to close most of their schools. For a listing of state site size policies, see www.cefpi.org/pdf/state_guidelines.pdf.

7. *Change grant criteria to encourage renovation over new construction.* In Massachusetts, the School Building Assistance Program provides "incentive percentage points" for school renovation/reuse proposals. Such points enhance a proposed project's prospects for state aid and encourage new school construction only when renovation is not feasible.

8. *Protect historic schools.* Pennsylvania policy states: "School districts should take all reasonable efforts to preserve and protect school buildings that are on or eligible for local or National historic registers. If, for safety, educational, economic, or other reasons, it is not feasible to renovate an existing school building, school districts are encouraged to develop an adaptive re-use plan for the building that incorporates an historic easement or covenant to avoid the building's abandonment or demolition" (www.nationaltrust.org/news/docs/20001018_award_pennsylvania.html). Historic schools taken out of service may be conveyed by school districts to nonprofit organizations and used for historic purposes for no remuneration.

9. *Provide dedicated funding for joint-use school projects.* California has passed two school bond measures (in 2002 and 2004), each of which dedicate $50 million to joint-use planning and construction. This funding supports the development of schools as integrated parts of their communities, around the colocation of child care centers, health clinics, libraries, and other public resources. The state legislature is also considering a bill that would expand the list of school construction projects currently eligible for joint-use funding to include parks, recreational centers, cultural arts centers, technology centers, health clinics, and athletic fields (www.nsbn.org/publications/newsletters/spring2004/hertzberg.php).

CHAPTER 5 LIST OF REFERENCES

[*This List of References is supplemented by a Master Resource List at the end of this PAS Report.*]

For general information on safe routes to schools programs go to:
- National Center for Safe Routes to School, www.saferoutesinfo.org/
- Transportation Alternatives, www.saferoutestoschool.org/

Beaumont, Constance. 2000. *Why Johnny Can't Walk to School.* Washington, D.C.: National Trust for Historic Preservation.

Bingler, Steven, Linda Quinn, and Kevin Sullivan. 2003. *Schools as Centers of Community: A Citizen's Guide for Planning and Design.* Washington, D.C.: National Clearinghouse for Educational Facilities. www.edfacilities.org/pubs/centers_of_community.cfm.

Ewing, Reid, and William Greene. 2003. *Travel and Environmental Implications of School Siting.* Washington, D.C.: U.S. Environmental Protection Agency. EPA231-R-03-004. October. www.epa.gov/smartgrowth/pdf/school_travel.pdf.

Goldberg, David. 2005. "Of Sprawl and Small Schools." *On Common Ground.* Winter. www.realtor.org/sg3.nsf/Pages/winter05sprawl?OpenDocument.

Gurwitt, Rob. 2004. "Edge-ucation." *Governing.* March. www.governing.com/textbook/schools.htm

Howley, Craig, and Charles Smith. 2000. *An Agenda for Studying Rural School Busing.* www.ael.org/rel/rural/pdf/busing.pdf#contents.

Hunter, Anna W., and Camille Sawak. 2003. *The Future of School Siting, Design and Construction in Delaware: Report and Recommendations.* Newark, Del.: University of Delaware Institute for Public Administration. July. www.ipa.udel.edu.

McClelland, Mac, and Keith Schneider. 2004. *Hard Lessons: Causes and Consequences of Michigan's School Construction Boom.* Beulah, Mich.: The Michigan Land Use Insitute. February. www.mlui.org/downloads/hardlessons.pdf.

Primer on School Planning and Coordination. 2002. Tallahassee, Fla.: Florida Department of Community Affairs, Division of Community Planning. www.dca.state.fl.us/fdcp/DCP/SchoolPlanning/Primergradcov.pdf.

Salvesen, David, and Philip Hervey. 2003. "Good Schools – Good Neighborhoods, The Impacts of State and Local School Board Policies on the Design and Location of Schools in North Carolina." Prepared for the Z. Smith Reynolds Foundation. Chapel Hill, N.C.: Center for Urban and Regional Studies, UNC-Chapel Hill. June. www.curs.unc.edu/curs-pdf-downloads/recentlyreleased/goodschoolsreport.pdf.

Toth, Mary E., and Wendy S. Kunz. 2003. "Guidelines for Establishing and Maintaining Community Partnerships for Better Schools, Better Communities, Better Opportunities, and Better Students." *Educational Facility Planner* 38, no. 4.

"*WHAT IF: Smart Schools.*" 2003. Los Angeles: New Schools Better Neighborhoods. www.nsbn.org/publications/whatif/2.php.

CHAPTER 6

Local and State Examples of Planning and Designing Active Communities

By Marya Morris, AICP, and Elaine Robbins

Since 2000, hundreds if not thousands of cities and counties have launched efforts to support active living. Planning and designing a physically active community is truly an interdisciplinary endeavor with more than a typical number of stakeholders, service providers, leaders, and decision makers. In every case, it requires a commitment of time, resources, and creativity on the part of elected officials, planners, and the public. The case examples profiled in this chapter are representative of what is happening across the U.S. Some efforts have been led by advocacy groups, such as WalkSanDiego and Feet First Seattle. In Portland, Oregon, and Ingham County, Michigan, the local and regional planning and transportation agencies, working in partnership with numerous other public agencies and community groups, have provided the catalyst for active living. In Denver, efforts to make the new urbanist community of Stapleton an active community have stemmed from a public private partnership among local developers, the city, and newly formed neighborhood groups. Underlying many of these initiatives has been the Active Living by Design (ALbD) program of the Robert Wood Johnson Foundation. The ALbD website (www.activelivingbydesign.org) contains descriptions of all 25 communities that received ALbD grants, including detailed information on the various approaches these communities and many others in the U.S. have put to use to create communities where residents can be physically active as part of their daily routine.

Sources for Denver Case Study

Forest City Enterprises Inc. 2004. Forest City Stapleton Web site. www. stapletondenver.com/main.asp

———. 2003. "Active Living Partnership Receives National Grant to Connect Health and Community Design at Stapleton." www.stapletondenver.com/news/press_detail.asp?pressReleaseID=53

DENVER, COLORADO

A major redevelopment project underway at Denver's old Stapleton International Airport offers an ideal template for putting active living ideas into action. Developers of Stapleton, the nation's largest urban infill project, hope to put 30,000 residents within walking distance of jobs, retail, schools, and public transportation. "We have a unique opportunity to develop 4,700 acres from the ground up," says Helen Thompson, chair of the Active Living Partnership at Stapleton. "The challenge is, Can you get it right from the get-go?"

In 2003, a consortium of public, private, and nonprofit organizations, led by Forest City Enterprises Inc., received a $200,000, five-year grant from the Robert Wood Johnson Foundation to promote physical activity in the Stapleton area. The consortium includes the University of Colorado Health Sciences Center, the City of Denver, the Stapleton Foundation for Sustainable Urban Communities, the Livable Communities Support Center, Feet First, Denver Healthy People 2010, and the Greater Park Hill Neighborhood Alliance to form the Active Living Partnership at Stapleton (ALPS). At the end of the five years, the Health Sciences Center will support the ongoing efforts of the Active Living program. "This diverse alliance of health and community design experts has tremendous potential to create model livable communities that promote active living and

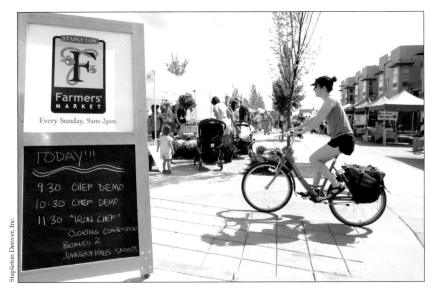

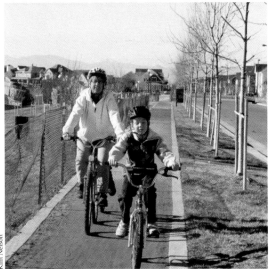

(Above) Most Stapleton residents ride a bike or walk to the local farmer's market each Sunday during the summer. (Left) A mother and son make use of the extensive trail system in the Stapleton community.

good health," said project supervisor Rich McClintock when the ALPS grant was announced.

The goal for the site is to build mixed-use, pedestrian-friendly, urban neighborhoods. Plans call for 12,000 homes ranging in price from $100,000 to $1 million, as well as low-income housing for seniors and apartments for a range of household incomes. In addition to housing and retail, the goal is for Stapleton to have 13 million square feet of offices and retail providing 35,000 jobs.

Now six years into a 20-year development, elements of the plan are starting to take shape. The developers have built about 3,000 units and one "town center" where residents can walk to restaurants, a supermarket, a café, and other stores. Residents of some of the surrounding existing neighborhoods—low-income areas that were long neglected in the shadow of the old airport—can also walk to the shopping area. "Before, the nearest grocery store was a couple of miles away," says Thompson. "Now it is right across the street."

Stapleton is 10 minutes from downtown Denver and 20 minutes from the new airport. To promote physically active lifestyles, the Active Living Partnership at Stapleton will encourage land-use and street design changes to promote safe walking and biking, conduct an outreach and incentives program for area businesses, and address barriers to physical activity around businesses and residences.

Stapleton is designed to offer the conveniences of urban living along with parks, trails, and walking paths. The commitment to smart growth has earned Stapleton international and national recognition, including the U.S. Conference of Mayors Public-Private Partnerships Award for Excellence and the Stockholm Partnerships for Sustainable Cities Award.

A citizens' advisory board is actively involved in the planning efforts, although some decisions have been controversial. Critics ask whether Quebec Square, a big-box retail center in another area of the vast Stapleton site that houses a Wal-Mart, Sam's Club, and Home Depot, fits the goals of a mixed-use, pedestrian-friendly development.

What's next on the drawing board? Planners are studying the best way to create bike and pedestrian connectivity between Stapleton and the adjacent town of Aurora. And plans for transit-oriented development include a multimodal station that will serve as a light rail stop connecting Stapleton to downtown and Denver International Airport.

Will all these efforts lead to more active and healthy living? "We won't know for a while yet whether people are more active," says Thompson. "We're making the best possible stab at it."

INGHAM COUNTY, MICHIGAN

Ingham County is home to Lansing, Michigan's capital, as well as East Lansing, the site of Michigan State University. In August 2004, the Ingham County Health Department published a report called *Our Health Is in Our Hands*, which presented the overall picture of health in the county.

According to the report, in 2002, inactivity was responsible for an estimated $8.9 billion in health-care costs in Michigan and $300 million in Ingham County alone. Although Ingham County's level of physical activity has improved since 1993, most residents do not exercise enough, and a quarter of the population is sedentary. Approximately 62 percent of Ingham County adults do not engage in moderate physical activity at least three times a week. However, almost 80 percent of Ingham County residents participate in some leisure-time physical activity. Leisure-time physical activity, according to Ingham County health officials, includes gardening or leisurely walking. County health officials hope that no more than 10 percent of county residents are inactive by 2010. To them, most

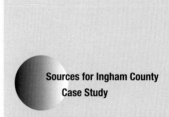

Sources for Ingham County Case Study

Capital Area Community Voices. 2004. CACVoices.org homepage. www.cacvoices.org

Capital Area Community Voices. 2004. "Land Use and Public Health." www.cacvoices.org

Glandon, Robert. 2004. Former Director of Planning and Special Services, Ingham County Health Department. E-mail interview with Marya Morris. September 14.

Ingham County Health Department. 2004. Our Health is in Our Hands. www.cacvoices.org

Tri-County Regional Planning Commission. 2004. Regional Growth—Choices for our Future. www.mitcrpc.org/pdfs/ Growth%20Project%20Library/ Tri-County%20Vision%20PE.pdf

people who engage in even low levels of physical activity will experience health benefits.

Population shifts over the past decade greatly affect the health of the county. Higher-income residents have moved in large numbers from the urban center to rural areas outside of Ingham County, which have experienced a boom in new home construction. At the same time, Ingham County, and particularly the Lansing/East Lansing urban center, has seen an increase in numbers of African-American, Hispanic, and foreign-born residents.

The shift has had health consequences for both groups, resulting in less active lifestyles for rural residents and declining health in the city. "Michigan is the most economically segregated state in the U.S.," says Bob Glandon, former director of planning and special services for the Ingham County Health Department. "This is causing a huge gap that is helping to exaggerate health disparities." African-American and low-income populations suffer much poorer health than the population as a whole. African-Americans in particular have higher rates of—and die earlier of—all of the top 12 medical conditions, including cancer, heart disease, birth defects, and diabetes.

Because of this, the health department hopes to do two things: make "health improvement" a goal of the master planning process at local and regional levels, and focus resources in geographic areas where health needs appear to be higher. An indicator used to determine areas with the greatest need is years of potential life lost (YPLL). Levels of health risks displayed by the population, such as smoking, substance abuse, poor diet, lack of exercise, and lack of access to health care, determine YPLL. Compared by census tract, the health department displays these results by map using GIS.

The health department used GIS to create a health impact assessment planning matrix that planners in 78 local government units can use to assess the impact of county development projects on health. The matrix enables planners to look at study the impacts in several categories, including water quality, wastewater disposal, air quality, solid and hazardous waste disposal, noise impacts, social capital, physical activity, and food systems. In terms of physical activity, questions asked include:

- Does the project provide mobility options for those who cannot drive?

- Does the project contain elements that enhance feelings of neighborhood safety?

- Does the project provide safe routes for children to walk to and from school?

- Does the project contain design elements to calm traffic?

- Does the project present unsafe conditions or deter access and free mobility for the physically handicapped?

- Does the project include pedestrian crossing signals and midstreet islands?

The health department held workshops for planners so they can begin to implement the matrix. A $12,000 grant from Michigan State University's Land Policy Program will fund this effort.

The tool still needs to be refined, according to Glandon. In the prototype phase, he says, "City of Lansing staff thought the tool could be good not only for evaluating individual projects but for master planning. But planners in some smaller jurisdictions—which have smaller staffs and fewer resources—said that for the tool to be useful, it would need to be simpler to use."

Another major initiative toward more active living is the Tri-County Regional Growth Project, supervised by the Tri-County Regional Planning Commission. This project is intended to actively engage citizens of the region to examine the implications of land-use trends and growth on the region's future. Ingham County, along with its neighbors Clinton and Eaton Counties, represent the Tri-County region in Michigan. Some of the regional themes and principles reflected in its policy map have been integrated into the comprehensive land-use plans of several local government entitites. Some of the principles that reflect land use and health include the following:

• The regional transportation priority will be to enhance and to preserve the existing road network, public transit, and nonmotorized transportation modes rather than further expansion of the road network in rural areas.

• Traditional neighborhood planning and design concepts (walkable elementary schools, mixed-use zoning, village/community design) will be implemented to maintain or reestablish viable neighborhoods, to attract new residents, and to eliminate impediments for existing residents to migrate to new developments.

• Pathways, sidewalks, trails, and on-street bike facilities should be developed and enhanced to provide alternatives to motorized transportation, to improve linkages to recreational opportunities for regional residents, and to provide public health benefits by offering opportunities for physical activity.

• Parks and recreation development and expansions should emphasize linkage of facilities through greenways based on the regional vision and the adopted Regional Nonmotorized System Plan.

The regional planning commission has set aside some money to fund projects that implement these goals, but funding is still a challenge. But sometimes help comes from unexpected sources. In 2004 the area became a nonattainment area for ozone, making it eligible for congestion air-quality money. Of those federal funds, $200,000 a year will be directed toward regional land-use projects that reduce emissions, encouraging healthy living in the process.

KING COUNTY (SEATTLE), WASHINGTON

Men's Fitness magazine named Seattle the fittest city in the U.S. in 2005. But while Seattle's residents hike in the mountains and lift weights in the city's many health clubs, they also spend a lot of time in the car. A 2004 study found that 58 percent of trips of less than a mile are made in a car. What's more, Seattle residents spend 35 percent more time stuck in traffic during peak times than in other hours.

This trend is troubling from a public health standpoint. The prevalence of obesity in the population more than doubled from 7 to 16 percent between 1987 and 2001. Obesity was responsible for about 15 percent of the deaths in King County in 1998 for adults over 18. Finally, deaths in King County from diabetes, which is often linked with obesity, have increased by more than 50 percent since the mid-1980s.

To address this trend, planners from the King County Department of Transportation are working with the health department and other partners on developing land-use policies that encourage active living. "When we started this project, the word 'health' was not even mentioned in the realm of land-use and transportation planning," says Don Ding, transportation project manager. "We are working to incorporate 'health' into key planning documents and actions."

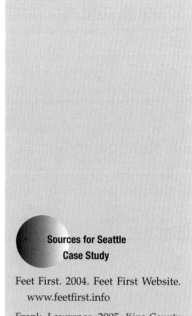

Sources for Seattle Case Study

Feet First. 2004. Feet First Website. www.feetfirst.info

Frank, Lawrence. 2005. *King County Land Use, Transportation, Air Quality and Health Study.* Seattle, Wash.: King County Department of Transportation. www.metrokc.gov/kcdot/tp/ORTP/LUTAQH/

Lawrence Frank & Company. 2004. *Achieving Sustainability Through Healthy Community Design.* Seattle, Wash.: King County Department of Transportation.

Rowe, Claudia. 2003. "Foot Soldiers in Push for Walkable Seattle." Seattle Post-Intelligencer, November 14. http://seattlepi.nwsource.com/printer2/index.asp?ploc=b&refer=http://seattlepi.nwsource.com/local/148316_feetfirst14.html

**PEDESTRIAN SUMMER
IN SEATTLE**

In 2003, Seattle held Pedestrian Summer, a campaign to promote walking and the safety of pedestrians. The campaign ran from May through "Walk to School Day" in early October. With the support of the city council, the mayor, city departments, community organizations, and businesses, the campaign fostered respect and civility between pedestrians and motorists and worked to improve driver behavior by increasing awareness about pedestrian safety. The city's long-term goal was to get people more excited about walking by creating a safer and more pedestrian-friendly cityscape.

The campaign demonstrated the city's commitment to walking as a vital mode of transportation, a healthy form of exercise, and a fun way to build community. The campaign tied together various public and private programs to encourage walking and pedestrian safety, in four components:

1. *Education*: providing information, presentations at public events, and mailings from insurance companies.

2. *Enforcement*: targeted enforcement by the Seattle Police Department of motorists who disobey crosswalk laws.

3. *Engineering*: new pedestrian safety devices installed by the Seattle Department of Transportation at troublesome intersections and school crossings.

4. *Encouragement*: guided walking tours and parade participation by pedestrian advocates and organizations.

Pedestrian Summer was awarded the Pedestrian Project Award for 2003 from the Institute for Transportation Engineers. For more information see www.pedsummer.org and http://www.ite.org/awards/pedproject/ppa062.pdf.

Source: Adapted from www.pedsummer.org

These efforts started in 2001, when King County initiated a study that would lead to smarter land development and transportation investment decisions. The King County Land Use, Transportation, Air Quality and Health Study (LUTAQH)—funded by a $350,000 Federal Transit Administration grant—identified how travel patterns, health, and overall quality of life are affected by specific land-use and transportation decisions within communities. The study examined the availability and quality of transportation that links residents to places of employment, recreation, entertainment, and other important destinations. The study noted: 1) how distance between activities affects residents' quality of life; 2) how mixes of land use stimulate walking; and 3) how residents feel about walking. For example, the amount of time spent walking between destinations can translate into improved public health. At the same time, the amount and distance that residents drive can cause regional air pollution.

The research team was led by Lawrence Frank & Company and included King County Federal Transit Administration, National Institutes of Health, the Center for Clean Air Policy, and the Puget Sound Regional Council. Research was conducted at the regional level, with more in-depth research for three case study communities: Kent Hill East, Redmond, and White Center.

The study found that more compact development, a wider variety of land-use mixes close to home and work, and more connected street networks with pedestrian facilities enhance walking opportunities. Walking increases as the numbers of retail and entertainment uses increase at the place of residence and employment. Finally, it found that street layout is an important predictor of travel behavior. Travel distance can be lower within a connected street network that enables walking.

A 2004 study, *Achieving Sustainability Through Healthy Community Design*, found that, on a per capita basis, residents of the most compact areas of the region generate 28 percent fewer vehicle miles than their suburban counterparts. Another finding shows that, as density increases to around 20 dwellings per acre, vehicle trips decline, while transit and pedestrian trips increase.

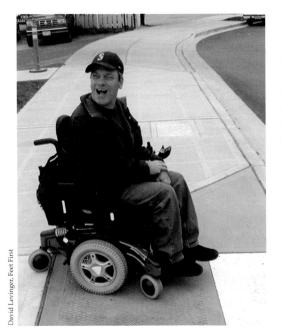

A wheelchair user road-tested new accessible sidewalks during a walkability audit of the Lake City neighborhood in Seattle, Washington.

David Levinger, Feet First

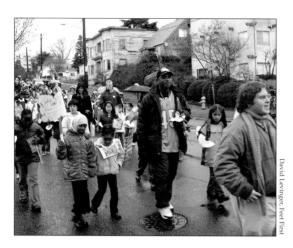

Students at Gatzert Elementary School in Seattle participating in a "March to School" on the Friday prior to Martin Luther King Day in 2006. The school also sponsors a Walking School Bus initiative.

David Levinger, Feet First

Seattle kids participated in a walkability audit in the city's Central District, using cameras to document crumbled sidewalks, obstructions, unsafe areas, such as parking lots with no pedestrian path markings, and places where improvements are needed, such as midblock crosswalks, new paved paths, and new signals.

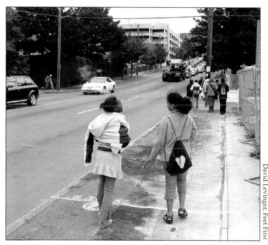

David Levinger, Feet First

The county is using findings from the two studies to create measures to make land-use and transportation investments more supportive of transit service and walking. Government agencies will illustrate the types of land-use and transportation actions that reduce auto dependence and promote walking and transit. After those steps are completed, the county will provide a series of recommendations for street network design and neighborhood compactness of development.

Another project to promote active living has been initiated by Active Seattle, a partnership between a nonprofit organization, Feet First, and the governments of Seattle and King County. Using a grant from the Robert Wood Johnson Foundation, the partnership is targeting five neighborhoods deemed in need of and receptive to pedestrian improvements: Greenwood, Delridge, Lake City, Beacon Hill, and the Central Area. Each of these neighborhoods ranges from 21,000 to 35,000 in population. Each neighborhood has a socioeconomic and racially diverse population, with Asians comprising between 12 and 51 percent, and African-Americans representing between 5 and 29 percent.

Feet First is promoting walkability in these neighborhoods through pedestrian maps, neighborhood maps indicating area assets, "walkability ratings," and stickers promoting an active lifestyle. The organization is also aiding sidewalk repair efforts. Feet First has also launched an Active Transportation initiative that has resulted in 16 years of state-dedicated transportation funding at $1 million to $2 million a year for Safe Routes to Schools.

But even in America's fittest city, it's sometimes easier to talk the talk than to walk the walk. Says Active Seattle project manager David Levinger, "The main challenge is prioritizing funding for these projects in competition with an aging highway infrastructure."

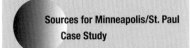

Sources for Minneapolis/St. Paul Case Study

Ernst, Michelle, 2004. "How Far Have We Come? Pedestrian Safety, 1994-2003." Surface Transportation Policy Project.

Hunt, Greg. 2003. "$200k Grant Awarded to County for Bike Trail." *Isanti County News*, November 19. www.isanticountynews.com/2003/november/19biketrail.html

Metropolitan Council. 2004. "Dates, Times Set for 'Walkable Community' Workshops in April." http://www.metrocouncil.org/directions/development/dev2004/walkable.htm

_____. 2004. *Transportation Policy Plan.* www.metrocouncil.org/planning/transportation/TPP/2004/summary.htm

_____. 2003. *The St. Croix Valley Development Design Study.* www.metrocouncil.org/planning/stcroixvalley/smartgrowth.htm

MINNEAPOLIS/ST. PAUL, MINNESOTA

A dilapidated strip mall in the Twin Cities Falcon Heights suburb is being transformed into a compact, pedestrian-friendly development called Falcon Heights Town Square. The centerpiece of the $35 million redevelopment project is a 120-unit apartment building that offers 10,000 square feet of street-level shops and businesses. Residents can walk to a city park, and bus service provides easy access to downtown Minneapolis and St. Paul, the University of Minnesota, and shopping hubs.

The project, designed to get people out of their cars, is just one of many supported by the Metropolitan Council, the regional planning agency of the Twin Cities metro region. The Metropolitan Council provided a $1 million grant that helped the city acquire the land for the Falcon Heights project and to make pedestrian improvements. The grant was offered through the council's Livable Communities Program, which promotes higher-density, mixed-use developments that offer good access to public transportation and amenities. Through this program, the Metropolitan Council offers grants to assist communities in connecting housing, retail, transit, and jobs.

The Twin Cities already ranks fourth among large metro areas on average annual spending per capita of federal funds on bicycle and pedestrian projects, according to a 2004 report from the Surface Transportation Policy Project. New Metropolitan Council programs, many related to transportation, support goals of improving multimodal transit. The latest transit improvement is the new Hiawatha light-rail line, which opened in 2004. Ridership on light rail exceeded expectations by 106 percent in its first year of operation.

In December 2004, the Metropolitan Council adopted a new Transportation Policy Plan that reflects a continued commitment to slowing growth in congestion, improving mobility, and providing transportation options. The plan calls for planning and investing in multimodal transportation choices; developing a network of dedicated rail and/or bus "transitways," including light rail; and encouraging local communities to implement a system of fully interconnected arterial and local streets, pathways, and bikeways. To reduce the need for single-destination car trips, the plan calls for encouraging mixed-use developments along transportation corridors.

The Twin Cities is one of the most nature-friendly areas in the U.S. according to the authors of *Nature Friendly Communities* (Island Press 2005). The book cited outstanding collaboration, sound regional planning, and a willingness to invest in resources to protect natural amenities. Since 1974, the Metropolitan Council has invested $367 million to help park agencies acquire and develop new parks and trails. The park system already has 52,000 acres and 170 miles of trails, and, in 2005, the Metropolitan Council adopted a policy that calls for the largest expansion of the regional parks and trails since the system was established in 1974.

In another move to promote active living, in 2004 the Metropolitan Council hosted walkable community workshops throughout the area. The workshops were designed for local elected officials, public administrators, health officials, transportation planners, and other local stakeholders. The workshops highlighted the ways in which local land-use and transportation decisions affect walking habits, personal health, and overall physical activity. During the four-hour sessions, local participants identified ways to reduce barriers to walking, to enhance opportunities for walking, and to build consensus on improving conditions for pedestrians and bicyclists. Examples generated in the workshops included creating neighborhood public centers (i.e. parks, open spaces), sidewalks, crosswalks, bike lanes, trails, traffic calming roadway design, public transportation, and housing near work.

As part of its effort to support smart growth, the Metropolitan Council has also been working directly with jurisdictions in the region to prepare smart growth plans. For example, in 2003 it prepared a study of the St. Croix Valley, a fast-growing area in the outlying reaches of the Metropolitan Council's jurisdiction. The *St. Croix Valley Development Design Study* addressed planned transportation improvements in the valley that the community and the Metropolitan Council anticipated would change travel patterns in the area and create pressure to develop newly accessible places. The goal of the design study was to shape growth in a way that is cost-efficient and appealing to taxpayers and local residents, and to give community leaders, citizens, and local government officials a chance to build a vision for how the St. Croix Valley should grow.

Recently, the Hennepin County public health department has gotten involved in the efforts to promote active living. In 2004 it launched an initiative to promote healthy living through community design. Hennepin County, which encompasses much of Minneapolis, faces such big-city challenges as poverty, crime, and an older infrastructure—all of which contribute to health problems. To address those challenges, the Human Services and Public Health Department joined with the Housing Community Works and Transit Department to form a community design committee. The committee met for a year and set several goals, among them: 1) to increase the daily physical activity level of county residents; and 2) to decrease injuries related to pedestrian, bicycle, and automobile collisions. The next step is to create a community design coalition that will develop a five-year plan to integrate healthy community design into all areas of planning in the county.

Another active living initiative is underway in Isanti County, a rural county due north of Minneapolis-St. Paul, which is another Robert Wood Johnson Foundation Active Living by Design grantee community. Isanti County is creating a multiuse trail corridor to connect the towns of Isanti and Cambridge. The trail project is being led by a consortium of city and county departments, including the Isanti County Parks and Recreation Department.

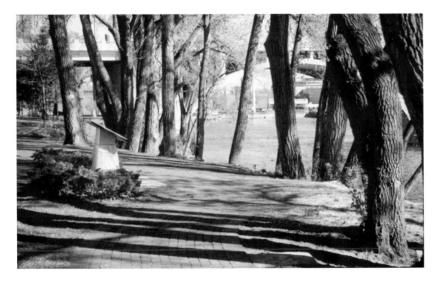

Researchers have found a strong correlation between the use of trails and the characteristics of the surrounding neighborhood. Specifically, trail traffic correlates positively and significantly with income, population density, education, the percent of neighborhood development in commercial use, the health of landscaping and vegetation, the amount of land devoted to parking, and block length (Lindsey et al. 2006).

This planned corridor will be the center of various activities that include a Safe Routes to School program and the creation of bike maps and signage for trail distances and points of interest. Nature loops along the trail will be included so the public has environmental and green space use along the path. This project will also conduct surveys gauging citizens' attitudes and behavior toward active living. The partnership with Active Living by

Sources for Nashville Case Study

Nashville Metropolitan Planning Department. 2003. *Metro Nashville-Davidson County Strategic Plan for Sidewalks & Bikeways*. www.nashville.gov/mpc/sidewalks/finalplan_march03.htm

Omishakin, Adetokubo. 2004. Music City Moves! Project Coordinator. Telephone interview with Marya Morris, September 7.

Design will include a marketing campaign and also serve as a model for promoting policy changes in a multijurisdictional setting.

If that's not enough to get people out of their cars, Congress's 2005 transportation bill should help. Minnesota was one of four states chosen to participate in a federally funded pilot program designed to ease traffic problems. The Twin Cities will get $25 million between 2005 and 2009 to build pedestrian and bike trails linking places where people live, work, and go to school.

NASHVILLE, TENNESSEE

Although Nashville has undergone an urban renaissance in recent decades, it lags behind other U.S. cities in designing a street and transportation network that encourages active living. Nashville has just half the mileage of sidewalks of comparable cities, and until 2000, bike lanes were practically nonexistent. As recent research has suggested, the absence of sidewalks results in an absence of walkers, which may be having a negative effect on the health of Nashville's residents. According to the Centers for Disease Control, Tennessee has one of the highest obesity rates in the country. *Men's Fitness* magazine gave Nashville poor marks for overweight/sedentary lifestyle and parks/open space in its 2005 ranking of "America's Fattest and Fittest Cities."

But that situation is starting to change. Thoughtful planning, use of public resources, and new regulations that require private developers to do their part reflect the city's new commitment to improving opportunities for daily physical activity. In one important step, Metro Nashville hired a group of consultants to create a plan for bicycle and pedestrian facilities. Completed in 2003, the *Metro Nashville-Davidson County Strategic Plan for Sidewalks and Bikeways* enables the area to plan for and implement facilities that improve safety, enhance mobility, and promote a higher quality of life. For fiscal year 2005-2006, $8 million was appropriated to implement the plan, which is expected to cost about $285 million over 13 years.

In terms of project coordination, three working committees participating in the planning process of the strategic plan. An Interagency Management Team monitored the progress of the planning process and was made up of representatives from the public works, planning, and finance departments, as well as the mayor's office. The team ensured coordination with city departments and quasi-public agencies whose work affects public rights-of-way. Finally, a Citizens Advisory Committee included individuals with interest or expertise in pedestrian and bicycle planning, neighborhood livability, disabled accessibility, public health, and urban design. Public input was obtained through public meetings, a telephone survey, website comments, direct correspondence, and a media campaign.

The main planning tasks included project initiation and data collection, evaluation of existing pedestrian and bicycling conditions, assessment of pedestrian and bicyclist needs, development of a proposed pedestrian and bicycle system, and development of design guidelines.

In terms of recommendations, the strategic plan provides a method for determining where sidewalks and other pedestrian improvements would maximize benefits. To meet this objective, a concept called the Sidewalk Priority Index (SPI) was created. SPI is intended to ensure that sidewalks are first constructed where existing need and potential for pedestrian traffic is the greatest, such as near schools, libraries, parks, and shopping centers. The methodology is based on a quantitative overlay system often used in regional environmental modeling. By overlapping a series of maps, each representing one of several characteristics, stakeholders can visualize the concentration of resources in a particular area. If each characteristic is assigned a number value (based on importance), the cumulative intensity of all characteristics in a particular area can be determined. SPI examines characteristics that most affect the potential of walking.

Also included in the recommendations section are design guidelines for pedestrian and bicycle facilities, as well as programs and special projects to increase alternate transportation. Steps have already been taken to raise awareness of new bicycle and walking opportunities among elementary aged children and seniors, and to educate them on ways to be safe while using them. Metro Nashville produced a guide that outlines requirements for property developers to fund sidewalks per the SPI.

After the completion of the strategic plan, the planning department received a Robert Wood Johnson Foundation Active Living by Design grant in late 2003. The department partnered with the Metro Public Health Department, Walk/Bike Nashville, and other organizations to form the Music City Moves! (MCM) partnership.

Partners are focusing on changing land-use policies and regulations at the county, city, neighborhood, and block levels to support physical activity. Another goal is to change the development practices of government officials and developers to include more opportunities for physical activity. To accomplish this goal, the planning department hired a land-use lawyer to review state and local planning laws to see which ones inhibit active living in communities. MCM also created an Active Living Neighborhood Audit Tool for Nashville communities. The results of these audits will be integrated into neighborhood design plans and used to achieve physical improvements as well as to provide information about what changes the public thinks are necessary.

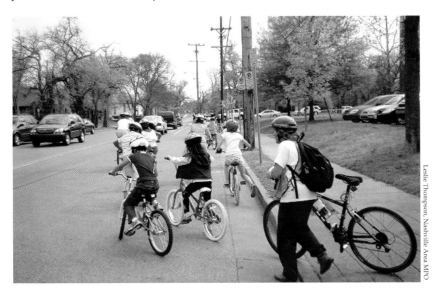

The Music City Moves Kids campaign in Nashville is modeled after the national Safe Routes to Schools program. MCMKids is one of three project in Nashville funded by a Robert Wood Johnson Foundation Active Living by Design grant.

Leslie Thompson, Nashville Area MPO

MCM has three main programs funded by Active Living by Design. As part of a $10,000 program called MCM Kids, the MCM partnership and community volunteers provided bike safety training and certification for school children. This program is modeled after the national Safe Routes to School program that started in California. The program also helped leverage funding for pedestrian improvements such as crosswalks and restriping along school routes. A program called Wise Moves, which had its kickoff event in summer 2005, encourages minority communities to use the stairs at work and to walk to lunch. The last program, Walk to Shop, will focus on improving active living for residents of a senior residential community in Nashville. The program leveraged government funds for physical improvements in the pedestrian

Tour de Nash is a walking and biking tour of downtown Nashville inaugurated in 2004. It was designed to introduce residents to available facilities and resources that support active lifestyles. Free blood pressure, cholesterol checks, body mass index measurements, and diabetes screenings are available on the day of the event.

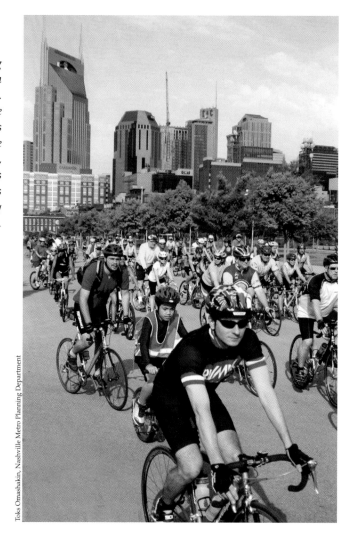

Toks Omashakin, Nashville Metro Planning Department

infrastructure near the senior residence. Plans are to create a walking club that encourages seniors to walk to shopping destinations such as grocery stores. MCM is working with Kroger grocery stores to allow walking club members to bring shopping carts to and from the senior center.

The partnership hired a public relations consultant to help coordinate special events to promote the local Active Living campaign. In May 2004, MCM hosted the inaugural Tour de Nash, a walking tour of downtown Nashville, a recreational bike ride, and free health and wellness screenings for blood pressure, cholesterol, body mass index, and diabetes. The other promotional campaign for 2004 was a weeklong event called Walk Nashville Week, which offered daily events for schoolchildren, seniors, and the general public.

MCM conducted educational sessions for policy makers, developers, and real estate professionals. Although there's still much to be done, the idea is starting to get out that a "livable city" is one that offers daily opportunities for active living.

PORTLAND, OREGON

Portland's decades of sprawl-busting efforts, its pedestrian-friendly downtown, and excellent light rail and streetcar system have made it a national model of land-use planning. That forward-thinking planning continues in efforts to encourage active lifestyles in the face of relentless development pressures.

Portland's Active Living by Design partnership promotes active living in three target neighborhoods. The partnership, led by the Oregon Coalition for Promoting Physical Activity and the American Heart Association Pacific Mountain Affiliate, is funded by a Robert Wood Johnson Foundation grant.

One project focuses on Damascus, a rural farming community that was incorporated into Portland's Urban Growth Boundary in 2003. Damascus is expected to urbanize rapidly over the next decade, and this project serves as a model of how to integrate active living principles in the initial stages of that growth. Damascus will be planned as a mixed-use community with an integrated system of streets, parkways, and greenways. The plan for the area addresses land-use, natural resources preservation, public facilities, and transportation. Newsletters, open houses, and other public events will ensure that the public has an opportunity to learn about the project and provide input. The study will create and evaluate concept plans for various uses and adopt plan designations that support those uses.

The second project was designed to increase use of walking, biking, and mass transit for daily transportation among the 3,300 residents of North Portland. The partnership sponsored activities and ideas for the Interstate Corridor Project to promote the new light rail line for the neighborhood. Planners used an individualized marketing program called TravelSmart to help residents improve their options for using light rail, walking, and biking for transportation. The first test run was from September 2002 to September 2003 in one Portland neighborhood. The program was designed with the following steps:

1. A "before" study used household surveys to determine travel behavior in a neighborhood.

2. Individualized marketing campaigns were directed towards households.

3. Two "after" studies—one six months after the intervention and one a year later—used household surveys to determine travel behavior after the completion of the marketing campaign.

The test run showed positive results. Vehicle travel miles were reduced by 12 percent, or 640,000 fewer vehicle miles traveled (VMT) per year. Travel by environmentally friendly modes increased by 27 percent. More specifically, public transportation increased by 27 percent, cycling increased by 40 percent, and walking increased by 32 percent. The gains in environmentally friendly modes of travel occurred across all age and gender groups and for all types of trips. Since the results support the use of TravelSmart as an effective strategy to increase environmentally friendly modes of travel and reduce car travel, the program will be used in other neighborhoods.

The third project targets Lents, a low-income community in southeast Portland. The project focused on improving access to the Springwater Corridor Trail, a recreational rail-trail that runs through the Lents community and is part of Portland's extensive trail network. "It's an extremely popular trail in the metro region, yet very few residents of Lents are aware that the trail exists in their community," says Noelle Dobson, project manager of Portland's Active Living program. Program leaders are promoting the trail and getting community and youth groups involved in trail improvements, including removing invasive species, planting trees, and removing trash. Long-term goals include building a trailhead in the community that will offer pedestrian and cyclist amenities.

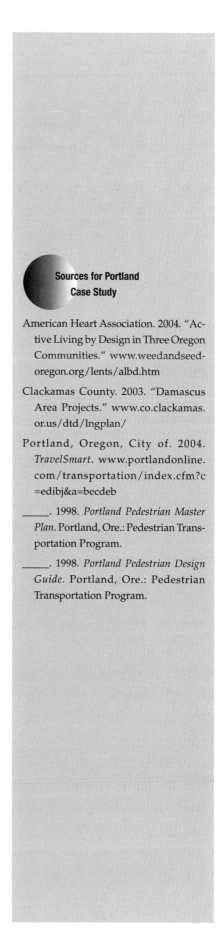

Sources for Portland Case Study

American Heart Association. 2004. "Active Living by Design in Three Oregon Communities." www.weedandseed-oregon.org/lents/albd.htm

Clackamas County. 2003. "Damascus Area Projects." www.co.clackamas.or.us/dtd/lngplan/

Portland, Oregon, City of. 2004. *TravelSmart.* www.portlandonline.com/transportation/index.cfm?c=edibj&a=becdeb

_____. 1998. *Portland Pedestrian Master Plan.* Portland, Ore.: Pedestrian Transportation Program.

_____. 1998. *Portland Pedestrian Design Guide.* Portland, Ore.: Pedestrian Transportation Program.

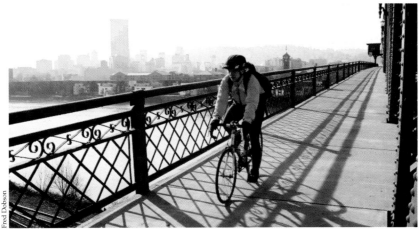

The bicycle commuter (above)
and the dog walkers (right)
shown here on the Willamette
riverfront and on a bike path
that crosses the river in Portland
are not part of an active living
program, rather they are just
making use of the city's excellent
infrastructure that supports
walking, bicycling, and transit.

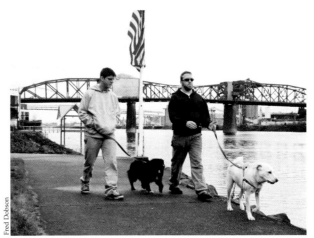

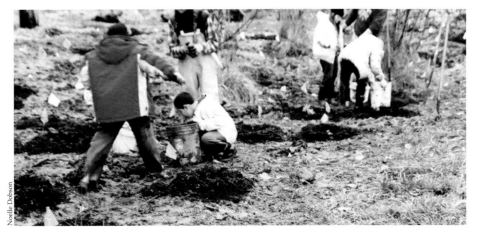

A trail-building session,
sponsored by Portland's
Active Living by Design
program, involved local kids
in planting trees along the
portion of the Springwater
trail that passes through their
neighborhood of Lents.

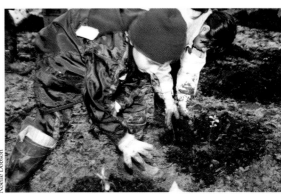

Portland's Office of Transportation continues to ensure that the city grows in a pedestrian-friendly direction. In 1998 it created the *Pedestrian Master Plan* and the *Pedestrian Design Guide*. The master plan was developed in accordance with the state Transportation Planning Rule (1991), which requires a reduction in vehicle miles per capita and changes to zoning and development codes to make them more pedestrian friendly. It also requires metropolitan areas/cities to adopt a transportation system plan with measurable goals aimed at increasing the modal share of pedestrian travel.

The master plan has a list of projects it recommends as needed improvements towards specific pedestrian facilities in the area. These recommended projects were selected through a sequence of actions that identified priorities. The first phase of actions involved assessing the needs of the pedestrian network in Portland and then coming up with a draft list of projects. Planners looked at the list of neighborhood needs regarding pedestrian facilities, conducted an inventory of sidewalks and curb ramps, plotted the locations of automobile-pedestrian crashes, and obtained feedback from communities regarding pedestrian needs in order to create the draft list.

Once the list was completed, the second phase involved selecting and creating a prioritized list of projects for the master plan. Each project on the draft list was assessed through a potential index and deficiency index. The potential index measures the strength of environmental factors used to justify a proposed project and whether these factors favor walking. The index includes policy factors, proximity factors, and environmental variables (e.g., land-use mix, destinations, connectivity, scale, and topography). Meanwhile, the deficiency index measures how many critical pedestrian improvements are needed within the location of the proposed project. Examples of critical improvements include replacing missing sidewalks, fixing difficult crossings, and providing connections where they are lacking.

The *Pedestrian Design Guide* integrates pedestrian design criteria and practices into proposed projects. It is used for all public and private development projects around the city. It includes guidelines for sidewalk corridors, street corners, crosswalks, pathways, and stairs. Over time, the integrated criteria will become the new standard in Portland, ensuring that the city continues to be a model of active daily living.

SAN DIEGO, CALIFORNIA

With near-perfect weather year-round and beautiful parks and beaches, San Diego is an outdoor recreation paradise. An active lifestyle is particularly easy for people who live downtown and in some of the nearby beach communities, which have pedestrian- and bike-friendly neighborhoods.

But some San Diego residents are spending more time in the car. Soaring housing prices—among the highest in the country—have forced many people to move to suburban communities, where they have long commutes and car-dependent lifestyles. As a result, San Diego ranks fourth among U.S. cities in time spent in traffic during peak periods, according to the Urban Mobility Report of the Texas Transportation Institute. To preserve the city's fit lifestyle in the face of such pressures, the San Diego Regional Planning Agency (SANDAG) and advocacy groups such as WalkSan Diego are working to promote physical activity in the county.

Two SANDAG programs in particular, the TransNet Bicycle Facilities Program and the Walkable Communities Demonstration Grant Program, have promoted active living. TransNet, a voter-approved initiative funded by a 0.5 percent countywide transportation sales tax, supports a variety of key transportation projects throughout the region. TransNet funding—$228

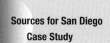

Sources for San Diego Case Study

Community Design + Architecture Inc., and W-Trans. 2002. *Planning and Designing for Pedestrians, Model Guidelines for the San Diego Region.* San Diego, Calif.: San Diego's Regional Planning Agency. www.sandag.org/uploads/publicationid/publicationid_713_3269.pdf

SANDAG (San Diego Regional Planning Agency). 2004. "TransNet Bicycle Facilities Program." Bicycle Facilities Program." www.sandag.org/index.asp?projectid=66&fuseaction=projects.detail

_____. 2004. "Walkable and Smart Growth Communities." www.sandag.org/index.asp?projectid=2&fuseaction=projects.detail

WalkSan Diego. 2004. "About WalkSan Diego." www.walksandiego.org/pages/about.html

million in 2005—is combined with state and federal dollars to improve San Diego's transportation network. The funding is distributed in thirds among highway, transit, and local road projects. Each year, $1 million is earmarked for bicycle facilities and programs. The TransNet Bicycle Facilities Program uses this money to help local agencies design and construct bicycle transportation facilities, install bicycle parking, and undertake bicycle safety and encouragement programs. It also improves the places where people bicycle and promotes cycling as a transportation option. There are currently 50 bicycle projects throughout the county.

When residents voted in 2004 to extend the TransNet Program, SANDAG increased the funding for bicycle and pedestrian projects to 2 percent of the total funding (approximately $4.5 million when the extension takes effect in 2009) and added a new expenditure plan called the Smart Growth Incentive Program. This program funds active living features such as pedestrian right-of-way improvements and denser development around public transit stations.

WalkSanDiego executive director Tina Zenzola explains to reporters plans to redesign University Avenue in North Park to more safely accommodate pedestrians and bicyclists. The plan was funded by a San Diego Association of Governments (SANDAG) Pedestrian Demonstration grant.

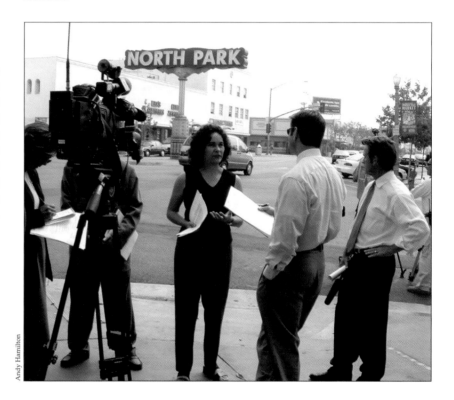

Andy Hamilton

The Walkable Communities Demonstration Grant Program was a one-time, $1 million program that used TransNet funds to show how a walkable community benefits neighborhoods, increases pedestrian safety, and contributes to smart growth planning. Through a competitive application process, SANDAG funded eight demonstration grant projects, which include streetscape improvement, crosswalk lighting, traffic calming strategies, downtown redevelopment planning, and street corridor improvements.

One demonstration grant project in the beach community of Encinitas has improved the streetscape of the downtown area. In the 1960s, the beach community's commercial district fell into decline when Interstate 5 was built and drew traffic and business away. Demonstration grant funds were used to install new crosswalks and improve landscaping and sidewalk buffers. These improvements build the recent historic preservation revitalization efforts of the Main Street Program, which earned Encinitas a Great American Main Street Award in 2004.

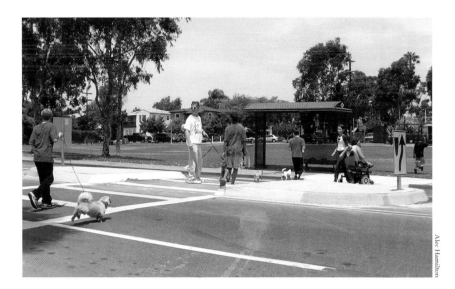

The crosswalk with pedestrian refuge island was designed by WalkSanDiego at the request of a local community group to provide safe access across a busy arterial street to the neighborhood's only park. The City of San Diego built the improved crosswalk.

An advisory committee on walkable communities was created in 1999 to provide SANDAG with advice on the walkable community demonstration grant program, as well as the walkability aspects of the smart growth strategies within the planning agency's comprehensive plan. The committee

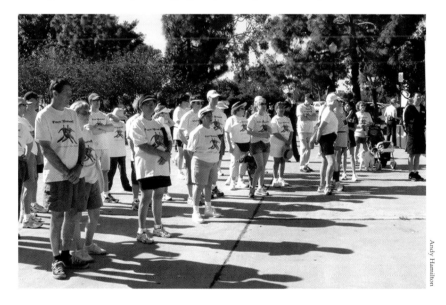

WalkSanDiego teamed with a local hospital to conduct a fitness walk in Balboa Park. Participants are shown here receiving instructions prior to the start of the walk.

included elected officials as well as public health and safety representatives, urban planners, engineers, academics, environmentalists, and community planning group representatives.

Also in June 2002, SANDAG created *Planning and Designing for Pedestrians, Model Guidelines for the San Diego Region.* This guide serves as a model for communities looking to create a more pedestrian-friendly environment. Topics include design recommendations for streets, walkways, accessibility, parking, and community structure that encourage the development of a walkable environment. SANDAG staff presented this information to the City of San Diego. The city has since modified its street design manual with wider sidewalks, buffers such as parkways and bike racks, and a new section on traffic calming. SANDAG continues to encourage the adoption of the guidelines into local ordinances or standards.

An organization that has successfully leveraged SANDAG funding is WalkSanDiego. This organization was formed in 1998 to enhance the

Sources for Arizona Case Study

Arizona Department of Health Services. 2004. *Physical Environment Workgroup Summary*. May 19. www.hs.state.az.us/phs/oncdps/ opp/pdf/physicalenvironment-may.pdf.

_____. 2004. *Physical Environment Workgroup Summary*. June 28. www.hs.state.az.us/phs/oncdps/ opp/pdf/environment.pdf.

livability of communities through promotion, education, and advocacy, by making walking a safe and viable choice for all people. Besides working with SANDAG to establish pedestrian policies and funding sources (including the Walkable Communities Demonstration Grant Program), WalkSanDiego has conducted historic walks, traffic calming workshops, neighborhood "walk audits," and pedestrian presentations. WalkSanDiego has also assisted numerous neighborhoods to design pedestrian safety improvements and assisted San Diego State University on a seminal study showing that residents of walkable San Diego neighborhoods walked more and had a lower body mass index.

Although the county hasn't yet measured the health impact of these efforts, indications are that programs like the demonstration grant program are spreading the gospel of active living. For example, when SANDAG launched a new pilot Smart Growth Incentive Program, the planning agency received 34 applications for projects. "Agencies got money, did projects, and people around the region saw how those projects benefited those communities," says Stephan Vance, senior regional planner at SANDAG. "I think there's a lot of momentum right now within local jurisdictions to do these types of improvements."

STATEWIDE CASE STUDIES

Arizona

In 2004, the Arizona Department of Health Services Obesity Prevention Program conducted workgroup meetings to identify strategies for a plan to reduce obesity and chronic disease through physical activity and nutrition interventions. Out of the workgroups came the Arizona Nutrition and Physical Activity Statewide Plan that focuses on improving nutrition, increasing physical activity, and addressing the effects of community design on health to reduce the number of overweight and obese state residents. A consortium of more than 40 organizations and agencies focused on families/community, worksites, health care, the physical environment, and schools. The statewide plan contains objectives and strategies to engage planners to modify local land-use and transportation plans to create active communities and prevent obesity.

Currently, there are various workgroups meeting to discuss issues and strategies specific to a certain group. Workgroups are divided by the following: worksite, elementary school, family, health care, junior high and high school, physical environment, special needs, and community. The physical environment workgroup has already identified strategies that they would like to see be implemented. One involves city planners and health initiative organizations working together to develop "best practices" for local communities to design their healthy community. Ideally, they would develop criteria, requirements, and funds for new and existing communities to promote physical activity. Another strategy would be to create or find an audit community assessment tool/report card to be used and implement at the local level. All these strategies are still subject to review but show promise during the early stages of their program.

Florida

In February 2004, the *Governor's Task Force on the Obesity Epidemic* finalized a report of its findings, as well as recommendations for the state. Overall, there were 22 task force recommendations, with various social units having a role in enforcing these recommendations. These units are community, family, healthcare providers, public health, schools, and worksites. The task force had two recommendations about planning the community to provide lifelong physical activity.

The first recommendation is for communities to promote access to lifelong physical activity opportunities by working with local governments, planners, land and real estate developers, organizations and associations, clubs, and other policy-making agencies within a specific community. Communities must review local environments and assess where improvements for physical activity opportunities may be implemented. Investment in bicycle and pedestrian infrastructure, review of transit-oriented development to promote walkable and bikeable communities, and review of long-term planning efforts to ensure that numerous physical activity options are available to residents for safe areas to exercise and play are also needed in Florida communities.

The second recommendation is for state and local agencies responsible for community planning to ensure that policies are routinely considered for accommodating pedestrians, bicyclists, and others who share the roadways and pathways in each community. These policies should also ensure that communities have bicycle and pedestrian development plans as part of their planning process for new construction. Agencies must also advocate for improved planning of new construction and determine the possibility of retrofitting current communities to designate safe areas for adults and children to exercise and play. This includes improvement for sidewalks, street lighting, traffic calming, and other environmentally safe constructs that encourage physical activity.

Keeping with the idea of ensuring accommodation for all who share the roadways and pathways, the Florida Pedestrian and Bicycle Program works to promote safe walking and bicycle through various programs. These include the Florida School Crossing Guard Program and the Florida Traffic Safety Education Program. The education program in particular focuses its efforts on local officials who tend to the needs of the public. Program deliverables includes pilot projects, research, media awareness campaigns, and the production of documents and guidelines.

Minnesota

A nonprofit organization, BeActive Minnesota, encourages physical activity through education and advocacy. BeActive Minnesota was formed in 2000 under a partnership between the Minnesota Department of Health, the Minnesota Council on Physical Activity and Sports, and the Minneapolis Heart Institute Foundation. The organization is most known for supporting various campaigns throughout the state. However, they also co-sponsor the awards of excellence program, which recognizes individuals, programs, and community groups that help improve the health of citizens in Minnesota through physical activity.

The state health department is also involved in a plan to creating a healthier environment. Called the *Minnesota Diabetes Plan 2010*, it seeks to promote policy change and improvements to the built environment as one of its goals. The plan hopes to accomplish this goal by identifying ways of increasing opportunities for physical activity and healthy eating, and by raising awareness among the public and policy makers about how the built environment affects health. Other steps include:

- changing existing policies and zoning codes to encourage land-development patterns that make working, shopping, going to school, and recreation possible within walking distance of where people live;

- promoting bicycling, walking, and other forms of physical activity as viable means of transportation; and

- ensuring that mobility needs are met by removing environmental barriers.

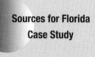

Sources for Florida Case Study

Florida Department of Health. 2004. *Obesity in Florida: Report of the Governor's Task Force on the Obesity Epidemic.* www.doh.state.fl.us/Family/GTFOE/report.pdf.

Florida Department of Transportation. 2004. "Pedestrian/Bicycle Safety Program Overview." www.dot.state.fl.us/safety/ped_bike/ped_bike.htm.

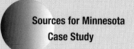

Sources for Minnesota Case Study

BeActive Minnesota. 2004. Home page. [Accessed July 9, 2004]. www.beactiveminnesota.org/

_____. 2004. "What We Need to Change." www.beactiveminnesota.org/about_change.asp.

Sources for New Jersey Case Study

New Jersey Department of Transportation. 2003. "New Jersey's Commitment to Bicycling and Walking." www.bikemap.com/RBA/.

New Jersey Pedestrian and Bicycle Resource Project. 2003. New Jersey Pedestrian Task Force homepage. http://policy.rutgers.edu/tpi/pedbike/force.html.

Sources for North Carolina Case Study

McArthur, Erica, et al. 2003. *Winning with ACEs! How You Can Work Toward Active Community Environments*. Raleigh, N.C.: Department of Health and Human Services, Division of Public Health.

Physical Activity and Nutrition Unit. 2004. *Eat Smart, Move More . . . North Carolina Executive Summary*. www.eatsmartmovemorenc.com/esmm/esmm_exec-summary.pdf.

New Jersey

The New Jersey programs highlighted here are transportation and pedestrian strategies to increase physical activity. Phase One of the *Bicycle and Pedestrian Master Plan* was completed in 1995, and Phase Phase Two in 2005. Phase Two involved updating the goals from 1995, creating a preliminary inventory of existing bicycle facilities, providing a method of prioritizing locations for bicycle and pedestrian improvements, and developing a vision for goals and an action plan. The vision of the plan is for New Jersey to be "a state where people choose to walk and bicycle. Residents and visitors are able to conveniently walk and bicycle with confidence and a sense of security in every community. Both activities are a routine part of the transportation and recreation systems and support active, healthy lifestyles."

The action plan had three strategies to achieve the vision and goals of the master plan: (1) data collection and tracking, (2) planning and facility implementation, and (3) education, enforcement, and encouragement. Data collection and tracking involves the creation of the inventory and methods to prioritize improvements. The planning and facility implementation part involves revising both the master plan and the Municipal Land Use Law and the Municipal Site Improvement Standards on a regular basis, and developing bicycle/pedestrian plans at the local level that include traffic calming facilities. Finally, the education part of the action plan would involve a media campaign.

The New Jersey Department of Transportation also teamed up with the Voorhees Transportation Policy Institute at Rutgers University to create the *New Jersey Pedestrian and Bicycle Resource Project*. Activities of the project include a pedestrian task force, bicycle advisory council, and information clearinghouse and toolbox for communities. The pedestrian task force is a state advisory group of professionals, advocates, and interested citizens who support walking as a safe, convenient, and sustainable form of transportation that increases the state's livability, enhances public life, and improves public and environmental health. They do this through education, collaboration, policy, activism, and advocacy. The task force has supported the International Walk to School Day in New Jersey, TEA-21 Reauthorization (alongside the New Jersey Bicycle Advisory Council), and a letter to the governor seeking support of bicycle and pedestrian friendly policies, projects, and funding.

North Carolina

In 2003, the North Carolina Cardiovascular Program published *Winning with Active Community Environments!*, a policy guide funded by the Centers of Disease Control and Prevention. The policy guide is a primer to creating the active community through public policy. The intended audiences include public health practitioners and their partners, grassroots community groups, and any interested individuals. The guide describes the history of land use and walkability, the planning agencies and resources that influence change, the ways to influence plans and policy statements to promote bike/pedestrian activity, the way to work with communities and the media, and the tools needed to assess existing infrastructure.

Two important documents that come from the policy guide include a community assessment and a worksheet on who makes decisions. The community assessment is a way to collect data and measure progress over time on how a community in North Carolina is doing in terms of promoting physical activity. Answers to questions have designated points, with the overall points determining how well a community is doing (higher point totals mean progress). The hope is that communities who self-assess and find their overall point total low will then make an effort to change their policies. Document number two, the worksheet on who makes decisions, acts as a sheet for communities to fill out in order to determine which people can influence change, which people can make governmental decisions, and when do all these people meet.

The organization in charge of distributing the policy guide is the *Eat Smart, Move More . . . North Carolina* initiative. The initiative is staffed by members of the Physical Activity and Nutrition Unit of North Carolina's Division of Public Health. Its main goal is to promote increased opportunities for healthy eating and physical activity through policy and environmental changes interventions and enhanced public awareness of the need for such changes. It has supported many health programs and organizations in the state as well as giving qualifying communities grant money to support physical activity and healthy eating programs at the local level. The website also has a resource library and contact directories for public use.

Oregon

In February 2003, the Oregon Department of Human Services released a separate plan for nutrition and one for physical activity. Both plans were created under the program, A Healthy Active Oregon. The program teams with the Oregon Coalition for Promoting Physical Activity and the Nutrition Council of Oregon to promote daily physical activity and healthy eating through implementation of Oregon's State Plans.

One of the goals from the physical activity plan is to foster communities that promote daily physical activity. To do this, the plan suggests an increase in:

- the number of communities where transportation and land-use planning foster daily physical activity;

- community-based recreational facilities and physical activity programs; and

- collaboration among public and private sectors to promote land-use planning and community designs that support bicycling and walking.

The program also published *What Can You Do? Small Steps Can Make a Big Difference*. It lists activities that individuals, parents, and employers can undertake to create more opportunities for physical activity. The document also lists suggestions for architects, community and transportation planners, and community leaders and policy makers. For the architects and community and transportation planners, it suggests design for more accessible and safe transportation options. For community leaders and policy makers, it suggests considering public health impacts in policy decisions and prioritizing funding for farmers' markets and pedestrian/bicycle facilities.

Pennsylvania

In 2003, the Pennsylvania Department of Health and the Pennsylvania Advocates for Nutrition and Activity (PANA) created a *Nutrition and Physical Activity Plan*. The mission of the plan is to create a state where individuals, communities, and public and private entities share the responsibility for developing an environment to support and promote active lifestyles and access to healthy food choices. These opportunities are supported in the plan through recommended strategies and activities necessary for community-based interventions. In terms of the physical environment, the plan has a section focusing on policy and environmental changes. It also calls for the social-ecological approach to create the changes. Ideally, this approach will promote change in various societal levels: the individual, group, institution/organization, community and society/public policy.

PANA's mission is to build an environment that will support and promote active lifestyles and healthy food choices. It uses the statewide plan as a guide, and its efforts are through education, advocacy and evaluation of

---

Sources for Oregon Case Study

Oregon Coalition for Promoting Physical Activity. 2003. *A Healthy Active Oregon: The Statewide Physical Activity Plan.* www.dhs.state.or.us/publichealth/hpcdp/physicalactivityandnutrition/paplan.pdf.

Oregon Department of Human Services. 2003. *What Can You Do? Small Steps Can Make a Big Difference.* www.dhs.state.or.us/publichealth/hpcdp/physicalactivityandnutrition/moore.pdf.

Sources for Pennsylvania Case Study

Pennsylvania Advocates for Nutrition and Activity. 2004. "Active Community Environments." www.panaonline.org/catmain.php?category=1.

Pennsylvania Department of Health. 2004. "Healthy Living for All Pennsylvanians." www.dsf.health.state.pa.us/health/cwp/view.asp?a=186&q=237170.

three areas: active community environments, youth and families, and health care. In terms of active community environments, its resource library has a plethora of information for the following categories: land use and transportation, recreation facilities/parks/trails, safety and security, and community and public health. Included in each category are information resources, tools and guides, technical assistance, data sources, related research, case studies, funding sources, and community-based programs.

Washington

The Washington State Department of Health created a *Nutrition and Physical Activity Plan* in June 2003. The executive summary of the plan summed up various dietary and physical activity guidelines for individuals. It also stated different indicators of the obesity epidemic: obesity rates have doubled over the last decade, half of all Washington State residents are obese, rates of chronic disease as disabling conditions associated with poor diet and lack of exercise continue to escalate year after year, and rocketing medical costs for obesity-related diseases are crippling Washington's ability to provide affordable health care coverage. Thus, the plan has objectives and priority recommendations specific to physical activity and nutrition. One of the objectives for physical activity is to increase the number of active community environments through planning, zoning, and land-use development, enlisting transportation policy and infrastructure changes to promote nonmotorized transit, and enhancing safety and perceived safety to improve community walkability and bikeability.

Besides the Department of Health, the Washington State Department of Transportation has supported various physical activity programs, including the statewide Walk to School and Bike to School programs. Updates to the Bicycle/Pedestrian Plan will be heavily influenced by the Nutrition and Physical Activity Plan. The Washington Coalition for Promoting Physical Activity, which supports individual and community solutions for increasing activity, has also turned out to be very influential in state efforts. Its members come from both the public and private sectors of the state.

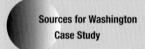

Sources for Washington Case Study

Washington Coalition for Promoting Physical Activity. 2003. "Physical Activity: It Fits With Life." www.beactive.org/index.html.

Washington State Department of Health. 2003. *Washington State Nutrition & Physical Activity Plan Executive Summary.* www.doh.wa.gov/Publicat/NPA%20Exec%20Summary.pdf.

Washington State Department of Transportation. 2004. Homepage. www.wsdot.wa.gov/.

CHAPTER 6 LIST OF REFERENCES

[*The resources used to compile the case studies in this chapter are listed in the sidebars adjacent to the case studies. These references are supplemented by a Master Resource List at the end of this PAS Report.*]

Lindsey, G., Y. Han, J. Wilson, and J. Yang, 2006. "Neighborhood Correlates of Urban Trail Use." *Journal of Physical Activity and Health* 3 (Supplement 1): S139–57.

Master Resource List

This resource list contains book, articles, and government document citations. The list is part of a continuous process and may be considered a literature review as well as a resource list for the project.

Texts were chosen for the resource list based on several criteria, including relevance to the topics of planning and the promotion of physical activity, timeliness, the ability to convey concepts accurately and concisely.

The resource list is arranged under the following topics:

- *popular literature:* material of interest but is not specifically about planning and physical activity, including articles that appeared in the popular press;

- *planning literature*: information written by/for planners;

- *health literature:* information written by/for medical and public health practitioners;

- *plans and guidelines*: outstanding plans and technical assistance documents from states and communities; and

- *law and legislation*: ordinances and other legal documents of interest.

This resource list will be updated regularly as new information becomes available. Additional web links and annotated descriptions of related web sites will be added continually.

Popular Literature

Brown, M. Gordon. 2001. "Healthy Sidewalks: A Guide for Property Owners." Space Analytics, LLC. July.

Burden, Dan. 2001. "Building Communities with Transportation." Distinguished Lecture Presentation. Washington, D.C.: Transportation Research Board.

California State Parent Teachers Association. 2001. *School Traffic and Pedestrian Safety Improvement: Resolution D*. Los Angeles.

California Safe Routes to Schools Initiative. 2000. *Safe Routes to Schools: Education, Engineering, and Enforcement for California Communities*. Sacramento: California Department of Health Services.

Chubb, Lucy. 2000. "Walking Trails Lead to Fitness, Study Says." *Environmental News Network,* March 18.

Engwicht, David. 1993. *Reclaiming Our Cities & Towns: Better Living with Traffic*. Philadelphia, Pa.: New Society Publishers.

_____. 1993. *Street Reclaiming: Creating Livable Streets and Vibrant Communities*. Philadelphia, Pa.: New Society Publishers.

Garcia, Gil. 2000. "Walkable Communities Initiative." *HopeDance Magazine* (September/October).

Jackson, Richard J., and Chris Kochtitzky. n.d. *Creating a Healthy Environment: The Impact of the Built Environment on Public Health*. Washington, D.C.: SprawlWatch Clearinghouse.

Kouri, Christopher. 1999. *Wait for the Bus: How Lowcountry School Site Selection and Design Deter Walking to School and Contribute to Urban Sprawl*. Charleston: South Carolina Costal Conservation League.

Moffett, Nancy. 2002. "Parks Stride Toward Fit City." *Chicago Sun-Times*, 22 March.

"Millions Have Obesity-related Syndrome." 2002. *Cnn.com/HEALTH*. Accessed October 28, 2002.

National Center for Chronic Disease Prevention and Health Promotion. 2002. "Promoting Physical Activity through Trails." Accessed October 28, 2002.

"A National Focus on Bicycling and Walking." 1994. *Transafety Reporter* 12 (September): 6-8.

O'Sullivan, Ellen. 2001. "Repositioning Parks and Recreation as Essential to Well-Being." *Parks & Recreation* 36 (October): 88-94.

Peirce, Neal. 2001. "Obesity and Sprawl: The Connection Tightens." *Washington Post Writers Group*. Accessed October 29, 2002.

Preservation Trust of Vermont. 2001. *A Local Official's Guide to Developing Better Community Post Offices*. Burlington, Vt.: The Trust.

Project for Public Spaces. 2001. "Health and Community Design."

Rails-to-Trails Conservancy. 2001. "Health Community: What You Should Know About Trail Building." Fact Sheet. 2001.

_____. 2001. "Trail Builders: What You Should Know About the Health Community." *Fact Sheet*.

Rudofsky, Bernard. 1969. *Streets for People*. Garden City, N.Y.: Doubleday Inc.

Sahagian, T. 1980. "Bicycle Commuting: It Makes More Sense than Ever." *Popular Mechanics* 153 (June).

Studemund, Gabrielle. 2001. "How to Grow a Sidewalk." *Cooking Light* (May): 43-44, 47.

U.S. Department of Agriculture Food and Nutrition Service. 2002. "10 Steps for Parents, Make Physical Activity Easy." *Fact sheet*. January. www.fns.usda.gov/tn.

Uhlman, Marian. 2000. "Communities Take Fitness Into Their Own Hands." *Philadelphia Inquirer*, February 21. www.communityinitiatives.com/article17.html (accessed October 28, 2002).

Vanderslice, Ellen. 2001. "Why Did the Pedestrian Cross the Road?: A Global Survey of Technical, Historical, and Philosophical Issues Around Crossing the Street." In *Writing the Wrongs*. S.l.: Women's Transportation Seminar.

Planning Literature

Appleyard, Donald. 1981. *Livable Streets*. Berkeley: University of California Press.

Beaumont, Constance E., and Elizabeth G. Pianca. 2000. *Historic Neighborhood Schools in the Age of Sprawl: Why Johnny Can't Walk to School*. Washington, D.C.: National Trust for Historic Preservation, 2000.

Bernick, Michael, and Robert Cervero. 1996. *Transit Villages in the 21st Century*. New York: McGraw-Hill.

Bicycle Federation of America. 1997. *Making America Walkable: The 1997 National Pedestrian Conference*. Washington, D.C.: The Bicycle Federation.

Bingler, Steven et al. 2003. *Schools as Centers of Community: A Citizen's Guide for Planning and Design*. Washington, D.C.: National Clearinghouse for Educational Facilities/KnowledgeWorks/CEFPI/Coalition for Community Schools.

Boarnet, Marlon G. 2004. *The Built Environment and Physical Activity: Empirical Methods and Data Resources*. Paper commissioned by the Transportation Research Board, Institute of Medicine. Committee on Physical Activity, Health, Transportation, and Land Use. www.trb.org/downloads/sr282papers/sr282paperstoc.pdf (accessed July 18, 2004).

Brown, Barbara B., and Vivian L. Cropper. 2001. "New Urban and Standard Subdivisions: Evaluating Psychological and Social Goals." *Journal of the American Planning Association* 67 (no. 4): 402–19.

Cervero, Robert and Roger Gorham. 1995. "Commuting in Transit Versus Automobile Neighborhoods." *Journal of the American Planning Association* 61 (no. 2) 210–24.

Conservation Law Foundation. 1998. *City Routes, City Rights: Building Livable Neighborhoods and Environmental Justice by Fixing Transportation*. Boston: The Foundation, June.

The Council of Educational Facilities Planners International. 2004. *Schools for Successful Communities: An Element of Smart Growth*. Scottsdale, Ariz.: The Council, September.

Crane, Randall. 2000. "The Influence of Urban Form on Travel: An Interpretive Review." *Journal of Planning Literature* 15 (August): 3–23.

Day, Kristin. 2003. "Urban Planning for Active Living: Who Benefits?" *Progressive Planning* 157 (Fall 2003): 1, 7–9.

De Cerreno, Allison L.C., and My Linh H. Nguyen-Novotny. 2006. *Pedestrian and Bicyclist Standards and Innovations in Large Central Cities.* New York: New York University, Wagner, Rudin Center for Transportation Policy and Management. January.

DeRobertis, Michelle. 2000. "Neotraditional Design: Mobility for All Ages." In *Urban Street Symposium: Conference Proceedings: Dallas, Texas, June 28-30, 1999.* Washington, D.C.: Transportation Research Board.

Does the Built Environment Influence Physical Activity? Examining the Evidence. 2005. Washington, D.C.: National Academies of Sciences, Committee on Physical Activity, Health, Transportation, and Land Use. Special Report 282.

Dolesh, Richard J. 2004. "Follow the Trail Toward Improved Health." *Parks & Recreation* 39 (May 2004): 40–46.

Donnelly, Steve, Yvonne Green, and Clacy Williams. 2004. *Collaborative Planning for Community Schools.* Fact sheet prepared for the 2004 American Planning Association National Planning Conference. Unpublished. April 27.

Duhl, L. 2002. "Health and Greening the City: Relation of Urban Planning and Health." *Journal of Epidemiology and Community Health* 56.

"Education and Smart Growth: Reversing School Sprawl for Better Schools and Communities." 2002. Translation Paper Number Eight. Miami, Fla.: Funders' Network for Smart Growth and Livable Communities. March.

Ernst, Michelle. 2004. *Mean Streets 2004, How Far Have We Come?* Washington, D.C.: Surface Transportation Policy Project.

Ewing, Reid. 1999. "Impacts of Traffic Calming." In *Urban Street Symposium: Conference Proceedings: Dallas, Texas, June 28-30, 1999.* Washington, D.C.: Transportation Research Board.

_____. 1999. "Mobility Friendly Street Standards for Delaware." In *Urban Street Symposium: Conference Proceedings: Dallas, Texas, June 28-30, 1999* . Washington, D.C.: Transportation Research Board, 2000.

_____. 1997. "Pedestrian- and Bicycle-Friendly Design." In *Transportation and Land Use Innovations.* Chicago: Planners Press, 1997.

Ewing, Reid, Otto Clemente, Susan Handy, Ross Brownson, and Emily Winston. 2006. "Identifying and Measuring Urban Design Qualities Related to Walkability." *Journal of Physical Activity and Health* 3: S223–S240. Supplement 1. Final Report available at http://www.smartgrowth.umd.edu/research/pdf/EwingClementeHandyEtAl_WalkableUrbanDesign_093005.pdf

Ewing, Reid, Christopher W. Forinesh, and William Schroeder. 2005. "Neighborhood Schools and Sidewalk Connections: What Are the Impacts on Travel Mode Choice and Vehicle Emissions?" *TR News* 237 (March-April). http://onlinepubs.trb.org/onlinepubs/trnews/trnews237environment.pdf (accessed December 29, 2006).

Ewing, Reid, and Robert Cervero. 2001. "Travel and the Built Environment: A Synthesis." *Transportation Research Record* 1780: 87–114.

Fenton, Mark. 2003. "Engineering Physical Activity back into Americans' Lives." *Progressive Planning* 157 (Fall): 12–17.

Forester, John. 1994. *Bicycle Transportation: A Handbook for Cycling Transportation Engineers.* Cambridge, Mass.: MIT Press.

Francis, Mark. 1999. *A Case Study for Landscape Architecture, Executive Summary.* Landscape Architecture Foundation, September.

Frank, Lawrence D. 2003. "Designing Communities with Health in Mind: The Basis for Effective Interventions." *Progressive Planning* 157 (Fall 2003): 36–37.

_____. 2000. "Land Use and Transportation Interaction: Implications on Public Health and Quality of Life." *Journal of Planning Education and Research* 20 (No. 1, 2000): 6-22.

Frank, Lawrence, and Peter Engelke. 2000. *How Land Use and Transportation Systems Impact Public Health: A Literature Review of the Relationship between Physical Activity and Built Form.* Atlanta: Centers for Disease Control and Prevention, Active Community Environments.

Frank, Lawrence, Peter Engelke, and Daniel Hourigan. 2000. *How Land Use and Transportation Systems Impact Public Health: An Annotated Bibliography.* Atlanta: Centers for Disease Control and Prevention, Active Community Environments.

Frank, Lawrence, Brian Saelens, and James Sallis. 2002. "Transportation Impacts on Human Health, Especially Physical Activity-DRAFT." Transportation Research Board. March.

Hall, Kenneth B., and Gerald A. Porterfield. 2001. *Community by Design: New Urbanism for Suburbs and Small Communities.* New York: McGraw Hill.

Handy, Susan. 2004. *Critical Assessment of the Literature on the Relationships Among Transportation, Land Use, and Physical Activity.* Paper commissioned by the Transportation Research Board, Institute of Medicine, Committee on Physical Activity, Health, Transportation, and Land Use. http://trb.org/downloads/sr282papers/sr282Handy.pdf

_____. 1996. "Urban Forum and Pedestrian Choices: Study of Austin Neighborhoods." *Transportation Research Record* (1996): 135–44.

Handy, Susan L., Robert G. Paterson, and Kent Butler. 2003. *Planning for Street Connectivity: Getting from Here to There.* Planning Advisory Service Report No. 515. Chicago: American Planning Association, May.

Hecimovich, James. 2004. "Linking School Siting and Land-Use Planning." San Francisco American Planning Association National Planning Conference Web Coverage, April 25.

Huang, Herman F., and Michael J. Cynecki. 2001. *The Effects of Traffic Calming Measures on Pedestrian and Motorist Behavior.* Report No. FHWA-RD-00-104. Washington, D.C.: Federal Highway Administration, August.

Jackson, L.E. 2003. "The Relationship of Urban Design to Human Health and Condition." *Landscape and Urban Planning* 64 (no. 4): 191–200.

Jaskiewicz, Frank. 2000. "Pedestrian Level of Service Based on Trip Quality." In *Urban Street Symposium: Conference Proceedings: Dallas, Texas, June 28-30, 1999.* Washington, D.C.: Transportation Research Board.

Killingsworth, Richard, and Thomas L. Schmid. 2001. "Community Design and Transportation Policies." *The Planning Journal: San Diego Chapter of the American Planning Association.* July.

Killingsworth, Richard, and Jean Lemming. 2001. "Development and Public Health: Could Our Development Patterns Be Affecting Our Personal Health?" *Urban Land* 60 (July): 12–16.

Kloster, Tom, James Daisa, and Rich Ledbetter. 2000. "Linking Land Use and Transportation through Street Design." In *Urban Street Symposium: Conference Proceedings: Dallas, Texas, June 28-30, 1999.* Washington, D.C.: Transportation Research Board.

Kreyling, Christine. 2001. "Hug That Transit Station." *Planning* 67 (January): 4–9.

Krizek, Kevin J. 2003. "The Complex Role of Urban Design and Theoretical Models of Physical Activity." *Progressive Planning* 157 (Fall): 28–29.

Kubilins, Margaret A. 2000. "Designing Functional Streets That Contribute to Our Quality of Life." In *Urban Street Symposium: Conference Proceedings: Dallas, Texas, June 28-30, 1999.* Washington, D.C.: Transportation Research Board.

Litman, Todd A. 2003. *Economic Value of Walkability.* Victoria, B.C.: Victoria Transport Policy Institute.

Lusk, Anne. 2003. "Designing the Active City: The Case for Multi-Use Paths." *Progressive Planning* 157 (Fall): 18–21.

Meyer, Michael D., and Eric Dumbaugh. 2004. *Institutional and Regulatory Factors Related to Nonmotorized Travel and Walkable Communities.* Paper commissioned by the Transportation Research Board, Institute of Medicine, Committee on Physical Activity, Health, Transportation, and Land Use. http://trb.org/downloads/sr282papers/sr282Meyer-Dumbaugh.pdf

Pisarski, Alan E. 1996. *Commuting in America II: The Second National Report on Commuting Patterns and Trends.* Lansdowne, Va.: Eno Transportation Foundation.

Pucher, John, and Lewis Dijkstra. 2000. "Making Walking and Cycling Safer: Lessons from Europe." *Transportation Quarterly* 54: 25–50.

Rietveld, P. 2001. "Biking and Walking: The Position of Non-Motorized Transport Modes in Transport Systems." In *Handbook of Transport Systems and Traffic Control.* Amsterdam: Elsevier.

Sallis, James F., et al. 2004. "Active Transportation and Physical Activity: Opportunities for Collaboration on Transportation and Public Health Research." *Transportation Research Part A* 38: 249–68.

Salvesen, David, and Philip Hervey. 2003. "Good Schools – Good Neighborhoods, The Impacts of State and Local School Board Policies on the Design and Location of Schools in North Carolina." Prepared for the Z. Smith Reynolds Foundation. Chapel Hill, N.C.: Center for Urban and Regional Studies, UNC-Chapel Hill. June.

Schimek, Paul. 2003. "City Planning: A Tool to Promote Physical Activity." *Progressive Planning* 157 (Fall): 30–31, 42.

Sclar, Elliott D., Mary E. Northridge, and Emily M. Karpel. 2004. *Promoting Interdisciplinary Curricula and Training in Transportation, Land Use, Physical Activity, and Health.* Paper commissioned by the Transportation Research Board, Institute of Medicine, Committee on Physical Activity, Health, Transportation, and Land Use. http://trb.org/downloads/sr282papers/sr282SclarNorthridgeKarpel.pdf.

Southworth, Michael, & Eran Ben-Joseph. 1997. *Streets and the Shaping of Towns and Cities.* New York: McGraw-Hill.

Ten Ways to Manage Roadway Access in Your Community. n.d. Tampa, Fla.: Center for Urban Transportation Research.

Terry, Carol. ed. 1986. *The Politics and Process of Urban Design: Stumbling Blocks or Stepping Stones: Seventh Annual Pedestrian Conference.* Boulder, Colo.

Toth, Mary E., and Wendy S. Kunz. n.d. "Guidelines for Establishing and Maintaining Community Partnerships for Better Schools, Better Communities, Better Opportunities, and Better Students." *Educational Facility Planner* 38, no. 4.

Transportation and Community and System Preservation Pilot Program. 2002. Washington, D.C.: Federal Highway Administration, U.S. Department of Transportation.

U.S. Environmental Protection Agency. 2003. *Travel and Environmental Implications of School Siting.* EPA 231-R-03-004. Washington, D.C.: U.S. EPA. October.

Vail, Kathleen. 2000. "A Piece of History: Districts Fight to Preserve Old or Historic School Buildings." *American School Board Journal.* http://www.asbj.com/lbd/2001/resources/102000vail.html (accessed December 29, 2006).

Warbach, John. 2005. "Bringing America Back in Sync with Its Values: Design Healthy Livable Communities Conference." *Planning & Zoning News,* January, 6–7.

Weihs, Janell. n.d. "School Site Size—How Many Acres Are Necessary?" *ISSUETRAK.* Washington, D.C.: Center for Educational Facilities Planners International. www.cefpi.org.

Wolshon, Brian, and James Wahl. 2000. "Planning and Design of a Suburban Neotraditional Neighborhood." In *Urban Street Symposium: Conference Proceedings: Dallas, Texas, June 28-30, 1999.* Washington, D.C.: Transportation Research Board, 2000.

Wright, C. L. 1991. "Urban Transport, Health and Synergy." *Transportation Quarterly* 45, no. 3.

Wyckoff, Mark A. 2002. "Health, Girth, Sprawl and the Great Lakes: Protecting Public Health and Safety Should Come First." *Planning & Zoning News*, January.

Zacharias, John. 2001. "Pedestrian Behavior and Perception in Walking Environments." *Journal of Planning Literature* 16 (August): 3–18.

Zegeer, C., and D. Feske. 1994. *Transportation Choices for a Changing America: National Biking and Walking Study.* Washington, D.C.: Federal Highway Administration.

Zelinka, Al, and Dean Brennan. 2001. *Safescape: Creating Safer More Livable Places through Planning and Design.* Chicago: Planners Press.

Health Literature

Abad, Ruth. 2005. "Making Healthy Choices, Easy Choices: Linking Health and the Environment. *Northwest Public Health.* University of Washington School of Public Health & Community Medicine. www.nwcphp.org/nph.

Aboelata, Manal J., et al. 2004. "The Built Environment and Public Health, 11 Profiles of Neighborhood Transformation." Oakland, Cal.: Prevention Institute. July.

Active Living Approaches by Local Governments. 2004. Washington, D.C.: National Association of Counties, November.

Active Living for a Lifetime: County and City Healthy Communities Profiles. 2006. Washington, D.C.: National Association of Counties, June.

Barton, Hugh, and Catherine Tsourou. 2000. *Healthy Urban Planning.* London: Spon Press on behalf of the World Health Organization.

Berrigan, D., and R. P. Troiano. 2002. "The Association between Urban Form and Physical Activity in U.S. Adults." *American Journal of Preventive Medicine* 23 (August): 74–79. Supplement.

Besser, Lilah M., and Andrew L. Dannenberg. 2005. "Walking to Public Transit: Steps to Help Meet Physical Activity Recommendations." *American Journal of Preventive Medicine* 29 (no. 4): 273–80.

Brownson, Ross C., and Tegan K. Boehmer. 2004. *Patterns and Trends in Physical Activity, Occupation, Transportation, Land Use, and Sedentary Behaviors.* Paper commissioned by the Transportation Research Board, Institute of Medicine, Committee on Physical Activity, Health, Transportation, and Land Use. http://trb.org/downloads/sr282papers/sr282Brownson.pdf.

Brownson, Ross, et al. 2001. "Environment and Policy Determinants of Physical Activity in the United States." *American Journal of Public Health* 91 (no. 12): 1,995–2,003.

_____. 2000. "Promoting Physical Activity in Rural Communities: Walking Trail Access, Use, and Effects." *American Journal of Preventive Medicine* 18 (no. 3): 235–41.

Buzbee, William W. 2003. "Urban Form, Health, and the Law's Limits." *American Journal of Public Health* 93, no. 9 (September): 1,395–99.

California Department of Health Services. 2004. "California Project LEAN [Leaders Encouraging Activity and Nutrition]." *Fast Facts.* October.

CDC (Centers for Disease Control and Prevention). 2005. "Barriers to Children Walking to or From School—United States, 2004." *Journal of the American Medical Association* 294: 2,160–62.

_____. 2004. "Health Risks in the United States: Behavioral Risk Factor Surveillance System." *At A Glance.*

_____. 2002. "Barriers to Children Walking and Biking to School – United States, 1999." *Journal of the American Medical Association* 288, no. 11 (September): 1,343–44.

Cervero, Robert, and Michael Duncan. 2003. "Walking, Bicycling, and Urban Landscapes: Evidence from the San Francisco Bay Area." *American Journal of Public Health* 93, no. 9 (September): 1,478–83.

Colditz, G.A. 1999. "Economic Costs of Obesity and Inactivity." *Medicine and Science in Sports and Exercise* 31: S663–S667. Supplement 11.

Cummins, S. K., and R. J. Jackson. 2001. "The Built Environment and Children's Health." *Pediatric Clinics of North America* 48 (October): 1,241–52.

Dannenberg, Andrew L., et al. 2003. "The Impact of Community Design and Land-Use Choices on Public Health: a Scientific Research Agenda." *American Journal of Public Health* 93, no. 9 (September): 1,500–08.

"Designing for Active Recreation." 2005. Research Summary. San Diego: Active Living Research. Updated February 2005. www.activelivingresearch.org.

"Designing for Active Transportation." 2004. Research Summary. San Diego: Active Living Research. January 2004. www.activelivingresearch.org.

"Designing to Reduce Childhood Obesity." 2005. Research Summary. San Diego: Active Living Research, February 2005. www.activelivingresearch.org.

Dora, Carlos. 1999. "A Different Route to Health: Implications for Transport Policies." 318 *British Medical Journal* (June): 1,686–89.

Drewnowksi, Adam, and Anne Vernez Moudon. 2005. "Fat Neighborhoods: Spatial Epidemiology Meets Urban Form." *Northwest Public Health.* University of Washington School of Public Health & Community Medicine. www.nwcphp.org/nph.

Dube, P. 2000. "Urban Health: An Urban Planning Perspective." *Reviews on Environmental Health* 15 (January-June): 249–65.

Duckhart, Jon. 2005. "Portland's Smart Growth Approach May Offer Health Benefits." *Northwest Public Health.* University of Washington School of Public Health & Community Medicine. www.nwcphp.org/nph.

Estabrooks, Paul A., Rebecca E. Lee, and Nancy C. Gyurcsik. 2003. "Resources for Physical Activity Participation: Does Availability and Accessibility Differ by Neighborhood Socioeconomic Status?" *Annals of Behavioral Medicine* 25 (no. 2): 100–04.

Ewing, Reid, et al. 2003. "Relationship between Urban Sprawl and Physical Activity, Obesity, and Morbidity." *American Journal of Health Promotion* 18 (September/October): 47–57.

Fraser, Barbara. 2001. "Documenting the Relationship between Physical Activity and Trails." PowerPoint Presentation from *TrailLink 2001 International Conference.* September.

Frumkin, Howard. 2005. "Health, Equity, and the Built Environment." *Environmental Health Perspectives* 113, no. 5 (May): A290–A291.

_____. 2005. "Urban Sprawl and Public Health." *Public Health Reports* 117 (May 2002): 201-217.

_____. 2005. "Ways Community Design Can Contribute to Health." *Northwest Public Health.* University of Washington School of Public Health & Community Medicine. www.nwcphp.org/nph.

_____. 2003. "Healthy Places: Exploring the Evidence." *American Journal of Public Health* 93, no. 9 (September): 1,451–56.

Geller, Alyson L. 2003. "Smart Growth: A Prescription for Livable Cities." *American Journal of Public Health* 93, no. 9 (September): 1,410–15.

Giles-Corti, Billie, and Robert J. Donovan. 2003. "Relative Influences of Individual, Social Environmental, and Physical Environmental Correlates of Walking." *American Journal of Public Health* 93, no. 9 (September): 1,583–89.

Goran, M. I., and M. S. Treuth. 2001. "Energy Expenditure, Physical Activity, and Obesity in Children." *Pediatric Clinics of North America* 48 (August): 931-53.

Guide to Community Preventive Services. 2003. "Promoting Physical Activity." *Fact Sheet.* www.thecommunityguide.org/pa/.

Handy, Susan L., et al. 2002. "How the Built Environment Affects Physical Activity: Views from Urban Planning." *American Journal of Preventive Medicine* 23 (August): 64–73. Supplement.

Healthy Community Design, Success Stories from State and Local Leaders. 2004. San Diego, Calif.: Active Living Leadership. December.

Healthy Places, Healthy People. Promoting Public Health and Physical Activity through Community Design. 2000. A Report of an Expert's Meeting, November 27-28. Washington, D.C. Sponsored by The Robert Wood Johnson Foundation.

Hoehner, Christine M., et al. 2003. "Opportunities for Integrating Public Health and Urban Planning Approaches to Promote Active Community Environments." *American Journal of Health Promotion* 18 (September/October): 14-20.

Humpel, Nancy, Neville Owen, and Eva Leslie. 2002. "Environmental Factors Associated With Adults' Participation in Physical Activity." *American Journal of Preventative Medicine* 22 (no. 3): 188–98.

Huston, Sara L., et al. 2003. "Neighborhood Environment, Access to Places for Activity, and Leisure-Time Physical Activity in a Diverse North Carolina Population." *American Journal of Health Promotion* 18 (September/October): 58–69.

The Interface of Urban Design, Public Health and Physical Activity in Preventing Obesity, December 2001 Conference. 2001. Seattle, Washington: Northwest Obesity Prevention Project, December.

Institute of Medicine. 2004. "Community Can Play a Role in Preventing Childhood Obesity." *Fact Sheet.* September.

Kaplan, Stephen, and Rachel Kaplan. 2003. "Health, Supportive Environments, and the Reasonable Person Model." *American Journal of Public Health* 93 (September): 1,484–89.

Killingsworth, Richard E., JoAnne Earp, and Robin Moore. 2003. "Supporting Health Through Design: Challenges and Opportunities." *American Journal of Health Promotion* 18 (September/October): 1–3.

Killingsworth, Richard E., and Thomas Schmid. 2001. "Community Design and Transportation Policies: New Ways to Promote Physical Activity." *The Physician and Sports-Medicine,* February.

King, A.C., et al. 2002. "Theoretical Approaches to the Promotion of Physical Activity: Forging a Transdisciplinary Paradigm." *American Journal of Preventive Medicine* 23 (August): 15–25. Supplement.

King, Wendy C., et al. 2003. "The Relationship between Convenience of Destinations and Walking Levels in Older Women." *American Journal of Health Promotion* 18 (September/October): 74-82.

Kirby, Susan D. and Marla Hollander. 2004. *Consumer Preferences and Social Marketing Approaches to Physical Activity Behavior and Transportation and Land Use Choices.* Paper commissioned by the Transportation Research Board, Institute of Medicine, Committee on Physical Activity, Health, Transportation, and Land Use. http://trb.org/downloads/sr282papers/sr282KirbyHollander.pdf.

Kohl, Harold and Karen Hobbs. 1998. "Development of Physical Activity Behaviors Among Children and Adolescents." *Supplement to Pediatrics* 101 (no. 3): 549–54.

Leyden, Kevin M. "Social Capital and the Built Environment: The Importance of Walkable Neighborhoods." *American Journal of Public Health* 25, no. 9 (September 2003): 1546-1551.

Librett, John J., Michelle M. Yore, and Thomas L. Schmid. 2003. "Local Ordinances that Promote Physical Activity: a Survey of Municipal Policies." *American Journal of Public Health* 93, no. 9 (September): 1399-1403.

Litman, Todd. 2003. "Integrating Public Health Objectives in Transportation Decision-Making." *American Journal of Health Promotion* 18 (September/October): 103–08.

Maantay, Juliana. 2001. "Zoning, Equity, and Public Health." *American Journal of Public Health* 91, no. 7 (July): 1,033–41.

Making Places for Healthy Kids: An Environmental Scan of Places Designed for Children to be Active. 2005. Seattle, Wash.: Active Living Network. February.

Maibach, Edward W. 2003. "Recreating Communities to Support Active Living: A New Role for Social Marketing." *American Journal of Health Promotion* 18 (September/October): 114.

McCann, Barbara. 2006. "Making Physical Activity Research Relevant to Policy Makers." *Journal of Physical Activity and Health* 3: S267–S272. Supplement 1.

McCann, Barbara, and Constance Beaumont. 2003. "Build Smart." *American School Board Journal* (October).

Moudon, Anne Vernez, and Chanam Lee. 2003. "Walking and Bicycling: An Evaluation of Environmental Audit Instruments." *American Journal of Health Promotion* 18 (September/October): 21–37.

Moudon, Anne Vernez, et al. 2006. "Operational Definitions of Walkable Neighborhood: Theoretical and Empirical Insights." *Journal of Physical Activity and Health* 3: S99–S117. Supplement 1.

Nestle, Marion and Michael F. Jacobson. 2000. "Halting the Obesity Epidemic: A Public Health Policy Approach." *Public Health Reports* 115 (January/February): 12–24.

Northridge, Mary E., and Elliott Sclar. 2003. "A Joint Urban Planning and Public Health Framework: Contributions to Health Impact Assessment." *American Journal of Public Health* 93, no. 1 (January): 118–21.

Orleans, C. Tracy, et al. 2003. "Why Are Some Neighborhoods Active and Others Not: Charting a New Course for Research on the Policy and Environmental Determinants of Physical Activity." *Annals of Behavioral Medicine* 25 (no. 2): 77–79.

Pate, R.R., et al. 1995. "Physical Activity and Public Health. A Recommendation from the Centers for Disease Control and Prevention and the American College of Sports Medicine." *Journal of the American Medical Association* 273: 402–07.

Payne, Laura, et al. 1998. "Local Parks and the Heath of Older Adults: Results of an Exploratory Study." *Parks & Recreation* (October).

Perdue, Wendy Collins, Lesley A. Stone, and Lawrence O. Gostin. 2003. "The Built Environment and Its Relationship to the Public's Health: The Legal Framework." *American Journal of Public Health* 93, no. 9 (September): 1,390–94.

Pollard, Trip. 2003. "Policy Prescriptions for Healthier Communities." *American Journal of Health Promotion* 18 (September/October): 109–13.

Powell, Kenneth E., Linda M. Martin, and Pranesh P. Chowdhury. 2003. "Places to Walk: Convenience and Regular Physical Activity." *American Journal of Public Health* 93, no. 9 (September): 1,519–21.

Pucher, John, and Lewis Dijkstra. 2003. "Promoting Safe Walking and Cycling to Improve Public Health: Lessons from the Netherlands and Germany." *American Journal of Public Health* 93, no. 9 (September): 1,509–16.

"Recommendations to Increase Physical Activity in Communities." 2002. *American Journal of Preventive Medicine* 22, no. 4S: 67–72.

Redman, L. 1999. "Neighborhood Safety and the Prevalence of Physical Inactivity – Selected State, 1996." *Center for Disease Control Morbidity and Mortality Weekly Report* 48 (February 26): 143–46.

"Research to Improve Children's Health." 2004. *Fact Sheet*. Describing findings from the Centers for Children's Environmental Health and Disease Prevention Research. Washington, D.C.: U.S. Environmental Protection Agency, November.

Romero, Andrea and Thomas Robinson. 2001. "Are Perceived Neighborhood Hazards a Barrier to Physical Activity in Children?" *Archives of Pediatrics and Adolescent Medicine* 155 (October): 1,143–48.

Saelens, Brian E., et al. 2003. "Neighborhood-Based Differences in Physical Activity: an Environment Scale Evaluation." *American Journal of Public Health* 93, no. 9 (September): 1,552–58.

Saelens, Brian E., James F. Sallis, and Lawrence D. Frank. 2003. "Environmental Correlates of Walking and Cycling: Findings from the Transportation, Urban Design, and Planning Literature." *Annals of Behavioral Medicine* 25 (no. 2): 80–91.

Sallis, James F., Adrian Bauman, and Michael Pratt. 1998. "Environmental and Policy Interventions to Promote Physical Activity." *American Journal of Preventive Medicine* 15 (no. 4): 379–97.

Sallis, James F., Katherine Kraft, and Leslie S. Linton. 2002. "How the Environment Shapes Physical Activity, A Transdisciplinary Research Agenda." *American Journal of Preventative Medicine* 22 (no. 3): 208.

Sallis, James F., et al. 2004. "Active Transportation and Physical Activity: Opportunities for Collaboration on Transportation and Public Health Research." *Transportation Research Part A* 38: 249–68.

Seattle/King County Public Health Department. 2002. "Overweight and Obesity in King County." *Public Health Data Watch* 5, no. 1 (March): 1–9.

Semenza, Jan C. 2003. "The Intersection of Urban Planning, Art, and Public Health: The Sunnyside Piazza." *American Journal of Public Health* 93, no. 9 (September): 1,439–41.

"Smart Growth Schools: A Fact Sheet." Washington, D.C.: National Trust for Historic Preservation. 2005. www.nationaltrust.org/issues/smart_growth.html.

Srinivasan, Shobha, Liam R. O'Fallon, and Allen Dearry. 2003. "Creating Healthy Communities, Healthy Homes, Healthy People: Initiating a Research Agenda on the Built Environment and Public Health." *American Journal of Public Health* 93, no. 9 (September): 1446–50.

Staunton, Catherine E., Deb Hubsmith, and Wendi Kallins. 2003. "Promoting Safe Walking and Biking to School: the Marin County Success Story." *American Journal of Public Health* 93, no. 9 (September): 1431–34.

Stokols, Daniel, et al. 2003. "Increasing the Health Promotive Capacity of Human Environments." *American Journal of Health Promotion* 18 (September/October): 4–13.

Sturm, Roland. 2005. "Childhood Obesity – What We Can Learn from Existing Data on Societal Trends, Part 1." *Preventing Chronic Disease: Public Health Research, Practice, and Policy* 2, no. 1 (January).

Sturm, R., and D.A. Cohen. 2004. "Suburban Sprawl and Physical and Mental Health." *Journal of the Royal Institute of Public Health* 118: 488–96. www.elsevierhealth.com/journals/pubh

Support for Walking, Biking, Trails, & Recreational Sites: Strategies to Promote Physical Activity in Nebraska. n.d. Lincoln, Neb.: Nebraska Department of Health and Human Services, Division of Health Promotion and Education.

Takano, T., K. Nakamura, and M. Watanabe. 2002. "Urban Residential Environments and Senior Citizens' Longevity in Megacity Areas: The Importance of Walkable Green Spaces." *Journal of Epidemiology and Community Health* 56, no. 12 (December): 913–18.

"THRIVE: Toolkit for Health and Resilience in Vulnerable Environments: Final Project Report Executive Summary." 2004. Oakland, Calif.: Prevention Institute, September.

Torres, Gretchen Williams, and Mary Pittman. 2001. "Active Living Through Community Design." In *Healthy People, Healthy Places.* Princeton, N.J.: Robert Wood Johnson Foundation.

"Trails for Life! Collaborative Promotes Rail Activity." 2003. The National Trails Training Partnership. May. http://www.americantrails.org/resources/health/trailsforlife.html

U.S. Department of Health and Human Services. 1999. *Promoting Physical Activity: A Guide for Community Action.* Champaign, Ill.: Human Kinetics.

_____. 1996. *Physical Activity and Health: A Report of the Surgeon General.* Atlanta, Ga.: U.S. Department of Health and Human Services.

U.S. Office of Disease Prevention and Health Promotion. 2001. *Healthy People in Healthy Communities: A Community Planning Guide Using Healthy People 2010*. Atlanta, Ga.: Office of Disease Prevention and Health Promotion.

"What's Health Got to Do with Growth Management, Economic Development and Transportation?" 2004. Seattle, Wash.: Puget Sound Regional Council, December. http://www.psrc.org/publications/index.htm#v2020issuepapers

Wilson, Rachel J. 2003. "Centering Suburbia: How One Developer's Vision Sharpened the Focus of a Community." *American Journal of Public Health* 93, no. 9 (September): 1416–19.

Plans and Guidelines

Aicher, Joseph. *Designing Healthy Cities: Prescriptions, Principles, and Practice*. Malabar, Fla.: Krieger Publishing Co., 1998.

Beatley, Timothy. 2000. "Bicycles: Low-Tech Ecological Mobility." In *Green Urbanism: Learning from European Cities*. Washington, D.C.: Island Press.

Bicycle Parking Facilities Guidelines. n.d. Portland, Ore.: The Office of Transportation. http://www.trans.ci.portland.or.us/Bicycles/parkguide.htm

Bikecentennial, Inc., and Bicycle Federation of America. 1993. *Balancing Engineering, Education, Law Enforcement, and Encouragement*. FHWA-PD-93-09. Washington, D.C.: Federal Highway Administration.

Burden, Dan, et al. 1999. *Street Design Guidelines for Healthy Neighborhoods*. Sacramento, Calif.: The Center for Livable Communities, January.

David Evans and Associates. 1992. *What Needs to Be Done to Promote Bicycling and Walking: National Bicycling and Walking Study: Case Study No. 3*. Washington, D.C.: Federal Highway Administration.

Daisa, James M., Tom Kloster, and Richard Ledbetter. 1998. *Does Increased Street Connectivity Improve the Operation of Regional Streets?: Case Studies from the Portland Metro Regional Street Design Study*. Portland, Ore.: Metro, 1998.

Della Valle, Beth. 2003. "My School Is a Smart Growth Honor School: State School Construction Policy." Presentation of the Maine State Planning Office at the State of the States on Smart Growth Conference, Burlington, Vt., October 9, 2003. www.maine.gov/spo/landuse/techassist/speeches/schools/index.php.

Emery, James, Carolyn Crump, and Philip Bors. 2003. "Reliability and Validity of Two Instruments Designed to Assess the Walking and Bicycling Suitability of Sidewalks and Roads." *American Journal of Health Promotion* 18 (September/October): 38–46.

Environmental Defense Fund. 1996. *A Network of Livable Communities: Evaluating Travel Behavior Effects of Alternative Transportation and Community Designs for the National Capital Region*. New York, N.Y.: The Fund.

Georgia Department of Transportation. 2002. *Pedestrian Facilities Design Guide*. Final Draft. December 20.

Gilbert, Richard, and Catherine O'Brien. 2005. *Child and Youth-Friendly Land-Use and Transport Planning Guidelines*. Toronto, Ont.: The Centre for Sustainable Transportation.

Gordon, Lavinia. 2003. "The Key to Good Health is Not in the Ignition: Portland, Oregon, Tries New Tool to Reduce Car Travel." *Progressive Planning* 157 (Fall): 4–5, 9.

Handy, Susan, et al. 1999. *Street Connectivity: A Report to the City of Austin on Cities with Connectivity Requirements*. Austin, Tex.: Community and Regional Planning Program, University of Texas at Austin.

Hexagon Group. 1996. *Plan for Parks and Recreation in Light Rail Station Communities*. Beaverton, Ore.: Tualatin Hills Park & Recreation District.

"Identifying and Measuring Urban Design Qualities Related to Walkability. Final Report." 2005. San Diego: Active Living Research, July.

JHK & Associates. 1987. *Planning and Implementing Pedestrian Facilities in Suburban and Developing Rural Areas: Research Report.* Washington, D.C.: Transportation Research Board.

_____. 1987. *Planning and Implementing Pedestrian Facilities in Suburban and Developing Rural Areas: State-of-the-Art Report.* Washington, D.C.: Transportation Research Board.

Local Government Commission. Center for Livable Communities. n.d. "Why People Don't Walk and What Planners Can Do About It." Sacramento, Calif.: The Commission.

Madison, Wisonsin. Traffic Engineering Division. 1997. *Pedestrian Transportation Plan for Madison, Wisconsin.* Madison, Wisc.: The Division.

"Making Schools Important to Neighborhoods Again." 2001. A Joint Report of the Maine State Board of Education and Maine State Planning Office to the National Resources Committee.

Maricopa Association of Governments. 1999. *Pedestrian Plan 2000.* Phoenix: The Association.

McGregor, Jennifer, and Todd W. Bressi. 2001. *WALKArlington: Places for Walking in the Rosslyn-Ballston Corridor.* Arlington, Va.: Arlington Greenway Core Working Group.

Metro Council. 2002. *Creating Livable Streets: Street Design Guidelines for 2040.* 2d ed. Portland, Ore.: The Council.

_____. 1998. *Metro 2040 Land-Use Code Workbook: A Guide for Updating Local Land-Use Codes.* Portland, Ore.: The Council.

_____. 1997. *Regional Framework Plan.* Portland, Ore.: The Council, 1997.

_____. 1997. *Urban Growth Management Functional Plan.* Metro Code. Title 6, Chapter 3.07. Portland, Ore.: The Council, 1997.

Morris, Marya. 1996. *Creating Transit-Supportive Land-Use Regulations.* Planning Advisory Service Report No. XXX. Chicago: American Planning Association.

New Jersey Department of Transportation. 1995. *Statewide Bicycle and Pedestrian Master Plan.* Trenton, N.J.: The Department.

Oregon Department of Transportation and Oregon Department of Land Conservation and Development. 1999. *Main Street When a Highway Runs Through It: A Handbook for Oregon Communities.* Salem, Ore: Oregon Department of Transportation.

Orlando, Florida, City of. 1998. "Transportation Element." In the *Growth Management Plan.*

Pedestrian Policies and Design Guidelines. 2005. Phoenix, Ariz.: Maricopa Association of Governments, April.

Pinellas County, Florida, Metropolitan Planning Organization. 1991. *Pinellas County Comprehensive Pedestrian Plan.* Clearwater, Fla.: The Organization.

Portland, Oregon, City of. Pedestrian Transportation Program. 1998. *Portland Pedestrian Design Guid .* Portland, Ore.: The Program.

Portland, Oregon, City of. Pedestrian Transportation Program. 1998. *Portland Pedestrian Master Plan.* Portland, Ore.: The Program.

"Prescriptions for a Healthy City." 2001. *Forum for Applied Research and Public Policy* 16 (Summer): 6–33.

Project for Public Spaces, Inc. 1998. *Transit-Friendly Streets: Design and Traffic Management Strategies to Support Livable Communities.* Federal Transit Administration, Transit Cooperative Research Program Report 33. Washington, D.C.: National Academy Press.

Rails-To-Trails Conservancy. 1998. *Improving Conditions for Bicycling and Walking: A Best Practices Report.* Washington, D.C.: The Conservancy.

RBA Group. 1996. *Pedestrian Compatible Planning and Design Guidelines.* Trenton, N.J.: New Jersey Department of Transportation.

Regional Transportation District. 1996. *Creating Livable Communities: A Transit-Friendly Approach.* Denver, Colo.: The District.

Santa Barbara, California. City of Santa Barbara's Transportation Planning and Alternative Transportation Web Site. http://www.santabarbaraca.gov/Resident/Transportation_and_Parking/Alt_Trans/Transportation Planning and Alternative Transportation

Shoshkes, Ellen, with Helga Crowley. 2004. *Planning and Designing a Community School to Promote Healthy Lifestyles.* Design Competition, Perth Amboy (N.J.) Public High School August

Suzan A. Pinsof Consutants. n.d. *Connecting People and Trails: Local Community Planning for Bicycling and Pedestrians.* Des Moines, Ia.: Iowa Department of Transportation, Iowa Trails 2000.

Transit-Supportive Land-Use Planning Guidelines. 1992. Ontario, Canada: Ministry of Transportation, Ministry of Municipal Affairs.

Transportation and Community and System Preservation Pilot Program Case Studies. Washington, D.C.: Federal Highway Administration, U.S. Department of Transportation. http://www.fhwa.dot.gov/tcsp/case10.html

University of North Carolina, Highway Safety Research Center. 1996. *Bicycling and Walking in North Carolina: A Long-Range Transportation Plan.* Raleigh, N.C.: North Carolina Department of Transportation.

WalkBoston. 1996. *Community Walking Resource Guide.* Boston: Massachusetts Highway Department.

Wallace Floyd Associates, Inc. 1998. *Massachusetts Pedestrian Transportation Plan.* Boston: Massachusetts Highway Department.

Washington State Department of Transportation. 1999. *Recommendations to Reduce Pedestrian Collisions.* Olympia, Wash.: The Department.

_____. 1997. *Pedestrian Facilities Guidebook: Incorporating Pedestrians into Washington's Transportation System.* Prepared by OTAK. Olympia, Wash.: The Department, September.

Wilkinson, Bill. 2000. *A Prescription for Active Communities: Objectives, Actions, and Indicators for Creating Bicycle-Friendly and Walkable Communities. DRAFT.* Bethesda, Md.: National Center for Bicycling and Walking. November.

Wisconsin Department of Transportation. 2001. *Wisconsin Pedestrian Policy Plan 2020.* Madison, Wis.: The Department, 2001.

_____. 1998. *Wisconsin Pedestrian Policy Plan 2020.* Madison, Wisc.: The Department.

Zegeer, Charles V., Cara Seiderman, et al. 2002. *Pedestrian Facilities Users Guide: Providing Safety and Mobility.* FHWA-ED-01-102. Washington, D.C.: Federal Highway Administration.

Law and Legislation

Albuquerque, New Mexico, City of. *Pedestrian Connections Provision.* Zoning Code, Chapter 14, Article 16.

Bellevue, Washington, City of. *Mid-Block Connections.* 20.25A.090 Perimeter Design District (E) Design Guidelines (2)(7).

_____. *Pedestrian Circulation and Amenities.* 20.25A.110 Design Review Criteria (A)(2).

_____. *Pedestrian Connections.* Bellevue, Wash. 220.25A.100 Downtown Core Design District (E) Design Guidelines (3).

Bend, Oregon, City of. *Shopping Center Parking Lot Connectivity.* 6 Section 24 (5) General Provisions—Off-Street Parking (g) Shopping Center Parking.

California, State of. *Safe Routes to School Construction Program.* California Streets and Highways Code, Sections 2331, 2333, and 2333.5.

Cambridge, Massachusetts, City of. *Bicycle Parking Requirements.* Article 6.000, Section 6.37.

_____. *Expanded Commuter Mobility Program Ordinance.* Ordinance 1139 (part), Section 10.17.040.

_____. *Municipal Vehicle Trip Reduction Plans Ordinance*. Ordinance 1139 (part), Section 10.17.170.

Clark County, Washington. *Circulation Plan*. Ordinance 12.05A.110.

_____. *Development Incentives*. 18.320.080.

_____. *Development Standards*. 18.320.070.

_____. *Pedestrian/Bicycle Circulation Standards*. Ordinance 12.05A.400.

Concord, North Carolina, City of. *Street Connectivity Requirements*. Article 10 Street Improvement Standards, Sec. 10.1.5 Street Connectivity Requirements. Unified Development Ordinance.

Eugene, Oregon, City of. *Bicycle Parking Standards*. General Standards for All Development. Sections 9.6000-9.6110.

_____. *Pedestrian On-Site Circulation*. General Standards for All Development 9.6730 Pedestrian Circulation On-Site.

_____. *Street Connectivity*. General Standards for All Development. 9.6815 Connectivity for Streets (1)(2).

Fort Collins, Colorado, City of. *Street Pattern and Connectivity Standards*. Article 3 General Development Standards, Division 3.6 Transportation and Circulation, 3.6.3 Street Pattern and Connectivity Standards.

Santa Barbara, California, City of. *Circulation Element*. General Plan.

Santa Cruz, California, City of. *Bicycle Parking Ordinance*. Section 24.12.250.

Seattle, Washington, City of. *Locational Criteria—Pedestrian District 1, P-1 Overlay*. Municipal Code, Section 23.34.086.

Web Resources

ACTIVE COMMUNITY ENVIRONMENTS
www.cdc.gov/nccdphp/dnpa/aces.htm

A CDC-sponsored initiative to promote walking, bicycling, and the development of accessible recreation facilities.

AMERICA WALKS
www.americawalks.org/

America Walks is a national coalition of local advocacy groups dedicated to promoting walkable communities. Members are autonomous grassroots organizations from across the country, each working to improve conditions for walking in their area.

CALIFORNIA SAFE ROUTES TO SCHOOL INITIATIVE
www.dhs.cahwnet.gov/routes2school/

One of the best state (or local) programs linking walking and schools.

CENTER FOR LIVABLE COMMUNITIES
www.lgc.org/center/

The Center for Livable Communities, a national initiative of the Local Government Commission (LGC), helps local governments and community leaders to be proactive in their land-use and transportation planning, and to adopt programs and policies that lead to more livable and resource-efficient land-use patterns.

COMMUNITY INITIATIVES
www.communityinitiatives.com

A consulting firm that promotes the Healthy Communities agenda.

CONSERVATION LAW FOUNDATION
www.clf.org/

The Conservation Law Foundation is the largest regional environmental advocacy organization in the United States.

INTERNATIONAL WALK TO SCHOOL DAY

www.iwalktoschool.org/

International Walk to School Day gives children, parents, school teachers, and community leaders an opportunity to be part of a global event as they celebrate the many benefits of walking. Last year, nearly 3 million walkers from 21 countries walked to school together for various reasons—all hoping to create communities that are safe places to walk.

NATIONAL CENTER FOR CHRONIC DISEASE PREVENTION AND HEALTH PROMOTION: NUTRITION AND PHYSICAL ACTIVITY

www.cdc.gov/nccdphp/dnpa/index.htm

A Centers for Disease Control and Prevention program.

NATIONAL CENTER FOR BICYCLING AND WALKING

www.bikewalk.org/

The National Center for Bicycling and Walking (founded as the Bicycle Federation of America) works for more bicycle-friendly and walkable communities. The NCBW offers information support, training, consultation services, and resources to public agencies, nongovernmental organizations and advocates, maintains the NCBW Resource Center, publishes the eNewsletter *CenterLines*, and a quarterly journal, *NCBW Forum*, and organizes the biennial Pro Bike/Pro Walk Conference and other special meetings.

NORTHWEST OBESITY PREVENTION PROJECT

depts.washington.edu/obesity/index.html

The Northwest Obesity Prevention Project was started in 1998 by a group of public health nutritionists. The mission is to establish and to support public health approaches to obesity prevention in the Pacific Northwest.

PEDESTRIAN AND BICYCLE INFORMATION CENTER

www.walkinginfo.org/

The PBIC is a clearinghouse for information about health and safety, engineering, advocacy, education, enforcement, and access and mobility.

RAILS-TO-TRAILS CONSERVANCY

www.railtrails.org/

The purpose of Rails-to-Trails Conservancy (RTC) is to enrich America's communities and countryside by creating a nationwide network of public trails from former rail lines and connecting corridors.

ROBERT WOOD JOHNSON FOUNDATION

www.rwjf.org/

The Robert Wood Johnson Foundation was established as a national philanthropy in 1972, and today it is the largest U.S. foundation devoted to improving the health and health care of all Americans.

SPRAWL WATCH CLEARINGHOUSE

www.sprawlwatch.org/

The Sprawl Watch Clearinghouse mission is to make the tools, techniques, and strategies developed to manage growth accessible to citizens, grassroots organizations, environmentalists, public officials, planners, architects, the media, and business leaders. The Clearinghouse identifies, collects, compiles, and disseminates information on best land-use practices.

TRANSPORTATION RESEARCH BOARD

www.trb.org/

The Transportation Research Board (TRB) is a unit of the National Research Council, a private, nonprofit institution that is the principal operating agency of the National Academy of Sciences and the National Academy of Engineering. The board's mission is to promote innovation and progress in transportation by stimulating and conducting research, facilitating the dissemination of information, and encouraging the implementation of research results.

WALKABLE COMMUNITIES, INC.

www.walkable.org/

A nonprofit corporation established in the state of Florida in 1996. It was organized for the express purposes of helping whole communities, whether they are large cities or small towns, or parts of communities (i.e., neighborhoods, business districts, parks, school districts, subdivisions, specific roadway corridors, etc.) become more walkable and pedestrian friendly.

MAKING GREAT COMMUNITIES HAPPEN

The American Planning Association provides leadership in the development of vital communities by advocating excellence in community planning, promoting education and citizen empowerment, and providing the tools and support necessary to effect positive change.

494. Incentive Zoning: Meeting Urban Design and Affordable Housing Objectives. Marya Morris. September 2000. 64pp.

495/496. Everything You Always Wanted To Know About Regulating Sex Businesses. Eric Damian Kelly and Connie Cooper. December 2000. 168pp.

497/498. Parks, Recreation, and Open Spaces: An Agenda for the 21st Century. Alexander Garvin. December 2000. 72pp.

499. Regulating Home-Based Businesses in the Twenty-First Century. Charles Wunder. December 2000. 37pp.

500/501. Lights, Camera, Community Video. Cabot Orton, Keith Spiegel, and Eddie Gale. April 2001. 76pp.

502. Parks and Economic Development. John L. Crompton. November 2001. 74pp.

503/504. Saving Face: How Corporate Franchise Design Can Respect Community Identity (revised edition). Ronald Lee Fleming. February 2002. 118pp.

505. Telecom Hotels: A Planners Guide. Jennifer Evans-Crowley. March 2002. 31pp.

506/507. Old Cities/Green Cities: Communities Transform Unmanaged Land. J. Blaine Bonham, Jr., Gerri Spilka, and Darl Rastorfer. March 2002. 123pp.

508. Performance Guarantees for Government Permit Granting Authorities. Wayne Feiden and Raymond Burby. July 2002. 80pp.

509. Street Vending: A Survey of Ideas and Lessons for Planners. Jennifer Ball. August 2002. 44pp.

510/511. Parking Standards. Edited by Michael Davidson and Fay Dolnick. November 2002. 181pp.

512. Smart Growth Audits. Jerry Weitz and Leora Susan Waldner. November 2002. 56pp.

513/514. Regional Approaches to Affordable Housing. Stuart Meck, Rebecca Retzlaff, and James Schwab. February 2003. 271pp.

515. Planning for Street Connectivity: Getting from Here to There. Susan Handy, Robert G. Paterson, and Kent Butler. May 2003. 95pp.

516. Jobs-Housing Balance. Jerry Weitz. November 2003. 41pp.

517. Community Indicators. Rhonda Phillips. December 2003. 46pp.

518/519. Ecological Riverfront Design. Betsy Otto, Kathleen McCormick, and Michael Leccese. March 2004. 177pp.

520. Urban Containment in the United States. Arthur C. Nelson and Casey J. Dawkins. March 2004. 130pp.

521/522. A Planners Dictionary. Edited by Michael Davidson and Fay Dolnick. April 2004. 460pp.

523/524. Crossroads, Hamlet, Village, Town (revised edition). Randall Arendt. April 2004. 142pp.

525. E-Government. Jennifer Evans–Cowley and Maria Manta Conroy. May 2004. 41pp.

526. Codifying New Urbanism. Congress for the New Urbanism. May 2004. 97pp.

527. Street Graphics and the Law. Daniel Mandelker with Andrew Bertucci and William Ewald. August 2004. 133pp.

528. Too Big, Boring, or Ugly: Planning and Design Tools to Combat Monotony, the Too-big House, and Teardowns. Lane Kendig. December 2004. 103pp.

529/530. Planning for Wildfires. James Schwab and Stuart Meck. February 2005. 126pp.

531. Planning for the Unexpected: Land-Use Development and Risk. Laurie Johnson, Laura Dwelley Samant, and Suzanne Frew. February 2005. 59pp.

532. Parking Cash Out. Donald C. Shoup. March 2005. 119pp.

533/534. Landslide Hazards and Planning. James C. Schwab, Paula L. Gori, and Sanjay Jeer, Project Editors. September 2005. 209pp.

535. The Four Supreme Court Land-Use Decisions of 2005: Separating Fact from Fiction. August 2005. 193pp.

536. Placemaking on a Budget: Improving Small Towns, Neighborhoods, and Downtowns Without Spending a Lot of Money. December 2005. 133pp.

537. Meeting the Big Box Challenge: Planning, Design, and Regulatory Strategies. Jennifer Evans–Crowley. March 2006. 69pp.

538. Project Rating/Recognition Programs for Supporting Smart Growth Forms of Development. Douglas R. Porter and Matthew R. Cuddy. May 2006. 51pp.

539/540. Integrating Planning and Public Health: Tools and Strategies To Create Healthy Places. Marya Morris, General Editor. August 2006. 144pp.

541. An Economic Development Toolbox: Strategies and Methods. Terry Moore, Stuart Meck, and James Ebenhoh. October 2006. 80pp.

542. Planning Issues for On-site and Decentralized Wastewater Treatment. Wayne M. Feiden and Eric S. Winkler. November 2006. 61pp.

543/544. Planning Active Communities. Marya Morris, General Editor. December 2006. 116pp.

For price information, please go to APA's PlanningBooks.com or call 312-786-6344.
You will find a complete subject and chronological index to the PAS Report series at www.planning.org/pas.